Dear Pamela + Norm

Get ready for a poo-poo-
spew explosion of the
most adorable kind.

SPOTLESS
BABY

Merry Christmas
+ get sleep while
you can!

Love
Therose
xxx

D1570668

Titles by
Shannon Lush and Jennifer Fleming
Spotless
Spotless 2
Speedcleaning
How to be Comfy
Save
Completely Spotless
Spotless A–Z

Title by
Shannon and Erin Lush
Kids Can Clean

Title by
Shannon Lush and Trent Hayes
Stainless

Title by
Jennifer Fleming and Anna-Louise Bouvier
The Feel Good Body

SPOTLESS BABY

Shannon Lush &
Jennifer Fleming

ABC
Books

The ABC 'Wave' device is a trademark of the
Australian Broadcasting Corporation and is used
under licence by HarperCollins*Publishers* Australia.

First published in Australia in 2015
by HarperCollins*Publishers* Australia Pty Limited
ABN 36 009 913 517
harpercollins.com.au

HarperCollins*Publishers*
Level 13, 201 Elizabeth Street, Sydney, NSW 2000, Australia
Unit D1, 63 Apollo Drive, Rosedale, Auckland 0632, New Zealand
A 53, Sector 57, Noida, UP, India
1 London Bridge Street, London, SE1 9GF, United Kingdom
2 Bloor Street East, 20th floor, Toronto, Ontario M4W 1A8, Canada
195 Broadway, New York, NY 10007, USA

National Library of Australia Cataloguing-in-Publication data:

Lush, Shannon, author.
  Spotless baby / Shannon Lush and Jennifer Fleming.
  ISBN: 978 0 7333 3409 2 (paperback)
  ISBN: 978 1 4607 0480 6 (ebook)
  Includes index.
  Housekeeping.
  Children – Health and hygiene.
  Other Creators/Contributors:
  Fleming, Jennifer, author.
640

Cover design by HarperCollins Design Studio
Front cover image: Baby boy getting messy eating spaghetti
by Quiet Noise Creative / Getty Images
Back cover image by shutterstock.com
Internal images by shutterstock.com
Index by Michael Wyatt
Typeset in Georgia by Kirby Jones
Printed and bound in Australia by Griffin Press
The papers used by HarperCollins in the manufacture of this book are a natural,
recyclable product made from wood grown in sustainable plantation forests.
The fibre source and manufacturing processes meet recognised international
environmental standards, and carry certification.

CONTENTS

Shannon Lush is a fine arts restorer and artist who uses a range of tools, adhesives and solvents to repair items. She has a deep passion for household handy hints, with knowledge passed down through her family. For the past decade, she's solved other people's domestic disasters though regular media appearances on radio and TV, and in newspapers and the best-selling *Spotless* series of books with Jennifer Fleming, as well as *Kids Can Clean* with Erin Lush and *Stainless* with Trent Hayes. She's never been stumped with a 'how to' question around the home and loves finding creative solutions to everyday domestic problems.

Jennifer Fleming is a long-time producer and presenter at ABC Radio working on a range of popular programs. She's also a best-selling writer of several books including the number 1 selling non-fiction title of 2006, *Spotless: room-by-room solutions to domestic disasters; Speedcleaning; How to be Comfy; Save: your money, your time, your planet; Spotless 2; Completely Spotless; Household Wisdom; and Spotless A–Z* with Shannon Lush. Her other books are *The Feel Good Body: 7 steps to easing aches and looking great*, with Anna-Louise Bouvier and *The Advertising Effect: how to change behaviour*, with Adam Ferrier.

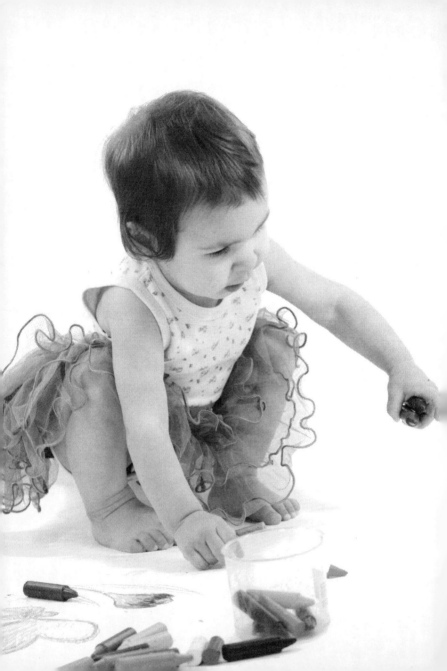

INTRODUCTION

Congratulations on your new bundle of joy. And welcome to your new life. Bringing a baby home for the first time is exciting and daunting for every parent. And while you've probably been told your life is about to be turned upside down, everyone's experience is different. You're about to begin a cycle of feeding, changing many nappies and washing mountains of clothes. And then there's the cleaning up. That's where we come in.

Spotless Baby tells you everything you need to know for safe, environmentally friendly and cost effective cleaning for babies to toddlers – from newborns to 3-year-olds. It includes advice on how to prepare your home for your new arrival, how to clean with baby in mind, how to sterilise items, how to select and store clothing, including hand-me-downs, and how to clean toys. It doesn't have any parenting advice, which may be a relief to you.

You've heard of a 'spring clean'. Get ready for the 'baby clean', a comprehensive and thorough cleansing of the home with tips on how to establish an efficient and low-fuss cleaning routine. There's advice on preventing stains while feeding and a comprehensive A–Z stain removal guide – from 'poo' to 'spew' and everything in between. You'll be happy to hear that the best cleaners are water and sunshine, with the sun naturally and safely fading many stains. Sunshine is also a chemical-free disinfectant.

Discover efficient bathing and changing routines, how to set up the baby's room and what to pack when leaving home on a short or long trip. There's even advice on how to deal with a 'poonami' – or poo explosion – and old-fashioned remedies passed down from generation to generation.

But it doesn't stop at your baby. There's plenty of advice on how to clean with one of the biggest creators of stains and mess – toddlers.

Help is at hand for this wonderful time of your life.

CHAPTER 1

SETTING UP HOME

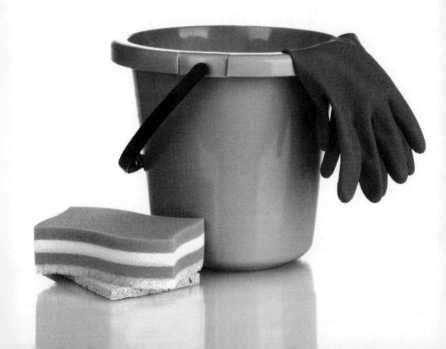

When a baby is on the way, your nesting instinct kicks in and with it comes a desire to get the house ready for your bundle of joy. In addition to clothing, a cot and a pram, you'll want to create a hygienic and organised home. We're not talking your regular clean or even a spring clean. It's 'baby clean' time.

CLEANING BEFORE BABY ARRIVES

A few months before the baby is due, take the opportunity to clean your home from top to bottom. Look at every room with a new set of eyes by lying on the floor at baby height. You might be surprised at the amount of dirt and fluff under beds, couches and cabinets. Make any repairs and get your cleaning kit organised – you're going to be very busy once bub comes home.

Debug your house

Long before your baby arrives, it's a good idea to fumigate your home, especially if there are pets or cockroaches around. When fumigating, you should leave your home for a couple of days and sleep elsewhere. If using commercial gels, apply them in advance so you can remove the gel before the baby is in the home. Cockroach baits take around 6 weeks to work. Avoid using aerosol insect killers around young children; they are safe for adults but not for children of any age.

According to *CHOICE Magazine*, **surface sprays** offer more long-term control. Apply to cracks, crevices and inside rubbish bins, cupboards, drawers and shelves. But make sure you don't spray surfaces on which food is handled. **Baits and traps** are also effective but shouldn't be used with surface or knockdown sprays because they contaminate baits and traps, making them ineffective. Use **knockdown sprays** when you see a cockroach.[1] Other cockroach remedies are available,

---

1 www.choice.com.au/reviews-and-tests/household/laundry-and-cleaning/pest-control/cockroach-killers-review-and-compare.aspx

but always handle with care. The Australian Pesticides and Veterinary Medicines Authority has an online portal where you can check whether a product has been approved for sale. Visit https://portal.apvma.gov.au/pubcris.

Make your own non-toxic cockroach deterrent by mixing 1 cup of uniodised salt, 1 teaspoon of lavender oil and 1 litre of water in a spray pack. Spray the solution around doors, windows, drains, air vents and areas where cockroaches lurk. It creates a barrier that cockroaches don't like to cross. Re-spray when you see cockroaches – more often during summer.

Once your home is debugged, clean every surface to remove all trace of insecticides.

 During pregnancy, you have much more fluid in your body. Drink more water, even if it means going to the toilet more often. Water is essential for the good health of your kidneys.

Problem:	**Aerosol stain/burn on hard surfaces**
What to use:	**White vinegar, cloth, sunlight, tea tree oil, brown bread**
How to apply:	The stain is from citronella oil used in aerosols. To remove, wipe with white vinegar on a cloth and expose to sunlight. For stains on wallpaper, wipe over the stain several times with 2 drops of tea tree oil in the centre of a slice of brown bread.

Floors and soft furnishings

Prepare to vacuum, mop and wipe. First up, ensure your vacuum cleaner is ready for the task. Clean the dust bag regularly and if bagless, clean the cylinder. If you have carpet, it should be thoroughly cleaned before the baby comes home. To do this, mix equal parts unprocessed wheat bran and bicarb and sprinkle over the carpet. Bran is an abrasive and bicarb is a deodoriser. Sweep the mixture into the carpet fibres with a clean broom. Leave for 5 minutes before vacuuming. Maintain your carpet by vacuuming once a week.

Shannon's DIY Carpet Steam-Clean

- Make sure windows are open for ventilation. Fresh air will also speed the drying time.
- Hire a carpet cleaner – available at supermarkets.
- Use half the amount of cleaning product that comes with the machine (saving the other half for later) and add 2 tablespoons of bicarb, 2 tablespoons of white vinegar, 2 tablespoons of methylated spirits, 2 teaspoons of glycerine and 2 teaspoons of eucalyptus oil. This is a great general cleaner so store it in a spray pack and use when needed.

Move furniture and clean behind and under it. For hard floors, sweep or vacuum in preparation for mopping. Shannon prefers to mop floors with a soft kitchen broom head stuffed down the leg of a pair of pantyhose. To secure it, tie the legs around the broom handle. Brooms are better than mops at getting into corners and can be rinsed under water more easily. As you mop, stand on an old towel and shuffle forward – you'll dry and polish the floor as you go. Use cold water on cork, wood, old lino or any absorbent surface. Other surfaces can withstand hot water, which helps to break down fats. Add 240 ml of white vinegar to the water to cut through dirt and grease and to make the surface non-slip. If there are dust mites, add 1 cup of black tea to the rinse water.

To clean soft furnishings, after vacuuming, put on thin disposable rubber gloves and wash your hands with soap and water in the sink. Lightly shake your gloved hands, move in front of the furnishing and rub over the surface with your gloved hands. Loose material, including pet hair, will transfer from the upholstery to the rubber.

Dusting and wiping

Each time you vacuum, clean dust from window sills or it will circulate into the room. Remove bacteria from high-touch areas such as light switches and door knobs by wiping with a cloth sprayed with 1 teaspoon of lavender oil in 1 litre of water in a spray pack. Lavender oil is a mild smell for babies. Don't use menthol or pine-based cleaners because they are harsh for a baby's lungs which are like little sponges.

Place a couple of drops of lemon oil on the head of a soft broom or a long-handled duster and dust ceilings and light fittings – the lemon oil will transfer to the dusted surface and inhibit spiders. Spray diluted lavender oil over flyscreens and check the screens are in good repair. If not, have them fixed. Wipe over door jambs and window frames with the lavender oil spray to deter bugs. Lavender oil is also antibacterial.

 TIP Check hinges and flyscreen door mechanisms – fingers can get caught. Place safety catches on cupboard doors.

Remove dust mites

Babies react more quickly to dust mites than adults so keep them to a minimum. When wiping over surfaces, add 1 cup of black tea to the wash water to kill mites. If vacuuming carpet, add 1 drop of lavender oil to a used tea bag and suck it into the vacuum cleaner. This will kill any dust mites inside the vacuum cleaner. Vacuum upholstered furniture and bedding – the most common areas for dust mites. Place 1 tea bag in 1 litre of cold water in a spray pack, allow it to steep for 3 minutes and lightly mist over surfaces. Spray on a cloth and wipe over pelmets, the tops of wardrobes and light fittings.

Air conditioners

If you have an air conditioner, clean the filter and trap every 2 weeks. Remove the pad and wash in the sink with a little dishwashing liquid. Dry in sunshine. The pad must be completely dry before being put back. Vacuum over the air conditioner vents and slats.

 TIP Place any toxic products out of reach, including detergents and cleaning powders. Keep items such as textas, pens, pencils and small items such as cotton buds and toiletries where your child can't reach them. To work out how high your child can reach, Shannon suggests giving them a piece of chalk and inviting them to draw on the wall. Store dangerous items above the highest chalk mark. Repeat each month – you'll be amazed at how quickly they grow and how agile they become. Chalk is easy to remove from walls.

Cleaning blinds

To clean cotton and fabric blinds, place 1 cup of unprocessed wheat bran in a large bowl. Add drops of white vinegar one at a time, stirring as you go, until the mixture resembles breadcrumbs. It shouldn't be wet. Place the mixture into the toe of pantyhose and tie it tightly. The tied section will be the size of a tennis ball. Wipe over the blinds as though using an eraser. When finished, store the 'bran ball' in a zip-lock bag in the freezer to use again. When vacuuming fabric blinds, stuff the vacuum cleaner head into the leg of a pair of pantyhose to prevent marks. To remove insect droppings, fill a 9 litre bucket with cold water and enough dishwashing liquid to generate a sudsy mix. Apply the suds only to the stains using a damp cloth. Rinse with a damp cloth.

When cleaning blinds, keep a clothes peg handy in case the doorbell rings or you get a text message. Peg the spot you're up to and you'll know where to resume cleaning.

Pets, especially cats, are a hygiene risk for babies. If you have them in the house, never allow them into the baby's room, regularly wash the pet and don't place your baby on the floor if the pet has been inside. Keep a doormat at each door to wipe your feet on, otherwise you'll track pet dirt and germs into the house.

How to get the most from your vacuum cleaner

The main elements of the vacuum cleaner are:

- **barrel:** this is the body of the cleaner. It has an inlet and outlet connection. The inlet is where the hose goes and it sucks dirt into the barrel. The outlet is where the air blows out of the machine and it's generally covered. You can attach the hose to the outlet to back-flush and clean the vacuum cleaner.

- **bag:** located inside the barrel. Modern vacuum cleaners have a window that shows when the bag is full. If you don't have this, check the bag each time you use the cleaner. It's a good idea to change the bag regularly. The vacuum cleaner won't work efficiently if the bag is more than half full.

- **tube:** the length of the hard part of the hose may be varied to suit your height or according to what you're vacuuming. Make it shorter when vacuuming furnishings and longer when vacuuming floors. If you are tall, extra lengths are available from the vacuum cleaner retailer or manufacturer and will save your back.

- **main head:** this can be set to have its bristles up or down. Vacuum with the bristles down for shiny and hard floors; put the bristles up for carpets and soft floors, unless you have pets. Clean any fur or dust out of the bristles with an old comb.
- **brush head:** a small, round attachment with long bristles designed to clean cobwebs, cornices, window sills, etc.
- **upholstery nozzle:** a small, flat attachment used to vacuum the surfaces of furnishings, curtains and pelmets.
- **corner nozzle:** used to access tight spaces, such as the sides of chairs, or to clean around the buttons on padded furniture.

 TIP Babies don't like the sudden noise of vacuum cleaners. Distract them with other sounds, such as the radio or TV.

How to keep mould at bay

Keep mould to a minimum because babies' respiratory tracts are still developing. Bleach only whitens mould – it doesn't kill it. Instead, wipe with ¼ teaspoon of oil of cloves in 1 litre spray pack of water on a cloth; don't spray directly. If wiping over walls, repeat every 6 months. Oil of cloves has a strong smell that's not dangerous but might disrupt the baby so wait until the smell dissipates.

The baby's room

Organise as much as you can before the birth because you're going to be busy when your baby comes home. Organise the room your baby will be sleeping in (it may be your bedroom), get clothes ready (washed and cleaned) and de-clutter as much as possible. Don't overdecorate the baby's room. You can add colours as they get older.

 If you have a fish tank, keep it clean to prevent algal bloom. Keep kitty litter boxes away from the baby's room because they are full of bacteria. If the litter box smells, it needs to be cleaned.

Five simple strategies to organise your home

Life in an organised home feels so much calmer, especially with a baby or toddler. But it's easy to go from clear to cluttered. One minute you can see the surface of your kitchen table; the next, it's covered in papers and other household items. The secret to an organised home can be summed up in one word – systems. Try these strategies and clear the clutter for good.

1. A place for everything, and everything in its place

No matter what the item is, everything – from scissors to socks – needs to have a designated storage spot. When you return items to their place, cleaning becomes speedier and life at home improves because you're not searching high and low for whatever you need. When working out where to store items, think about creating the smallest walking distance between two points – where items are stored and where they are used. For example, scissors could be kept in a kitchen drawer or in an office drawer, or you may decide to have two pairs if they are used often in both locations. You don't want to be constantly going backwards and forwards. For items that don't have a regular home, set up a 'miscellaneous' bowl or basket. Just make sure you clear it out regularly.

2. Do a little bit often
It's easy to let items pile up but you're just creating more work for yourself. Keep in mind that old saying: 'a stitch in time saves nine'. It's better to have one pile than nine. Schedule this task if you need to. You'd be surprised at how much you can do in just 15 minutes. Sort, file or toss.

3. Introduce the 'clutter bucket'
When sorting and tidying a room, everything that doesn't belong in that room can go into a 'clutter bucket' and moved in one go. It's common to move a couple of items at a time, with a lot of time – and energy – spent walking between two spots. Move items all at once with the clutter bucket. A regular 9 litre bucket is ideal for this.

4. Have the right cleaning tools for the job
It's important to have the right cleaning tools for the job. You might like to carry items in buckets or plastic toolboxes – it depends on your storage situation and preferences. Whatever you decide to use, just make sure the kit isn't too heavy. Keeping all your cleaning tools together means you won't waste time or put off cleaning because you don't have the right items. Your kit is always ready to go.

5. Maintain daily, weekly and monthly cleaning schedules
Make your life more organised and easy by creating daily, weekly
and monthly cleaning schedules. For example, if you clean the
oven once a week, you won't create a mega-task for yourself.
That baked-on gunk just gets harder to clean the longer you
leave it. A schedule – written and placed on the inside door in
the laundry, for example – will show you what needs to be done
and when.

How to make your pregnancy clothing expand with you

There was a time when pregnancy fashion meant tent dresses
with large bows. Fortunately, there are many more clothing
options available today but some are very expensive. It's easy
to add elastic to a pair of jeans or to adjust a couple of shirts.
See page 236 for more detailed instructions. You don't want
anything tight across your belly. Choose soft, stretchy fabrics.

Morning sickness remedies

80 per cent of expectant mothers experience morning sickness
but it's not only in the morning when a feeling of nausea can hit.
Before getting out of bed, drink a cup or tea and eat a couple
of dry biscuits. Because your body consumes more resources
when you're pregnant, you often wake up feeling hungry. Tea
and bikkies will help.

Other suggestions:

- For daytime sickness, eat a small spear of green pineapple.
- For afternoon sickness, drink ginger tea.
- Eat small meals regularly.
- When going out, take sick bags and find out the location of the nearest toilet. This saves being embarrassed in public. You'll need to pee more often so if you know where toilets are, you'll feel more secure.

 Many women have swollen ankles during pregnancy. If yours swell up, tell your doctor.

 Before your baby arrives, work out the best takeaway options near you and keep the list handy.

BABY EQUIPMENT

You'll need a range of baby equipment. Some will be bought new, other items passed on or bought second hand. If buying second hand, the Australian Competition and Consumer Commission (ACCC) suggests you only buy items that include full instructions (or check for instructions online). Make sure the item is sturdy and stable, has no missing parts, works correctly, has no tears, sharp edges or sharp points, has had no changes made that could make it unsafe, such as the wrong size mattress in a cot, or has had rough, non-professional repairs. If it doesn't meet these standards, don't buy it.

How to choose a baby capsule or child car restraint

You'll need a capsule to bring your baby home from hospital and when travelling in a car. Many parents rent one rather than buy. In cars, children under 6 months must be in an approved rear-facing child restraint with an approved anchorage system. If possible, have restraints fitted at an approved fitting station. Contact your local road traffic authority or Kidsafe for locations.

According to *CHOICE Magazine*, child car restraints must have a tether strap and five-point harness with a single-point adjustment and quick-release buckle. Each seat must be subjected to performance tests that simulate front, side and rear impacts, and come with instructions about installation, use and maintenance and general information. There's also a range of warning statements that must be permanently and legibly marked on the restraint.[2]

In Australia in 2014, the Child Restraint Evaluation Program (CREP) issued these legal requirements:

- Children up to the age of 6 months must be secured in an approved rearward-facing restraint.
- Children aged from 6 months old but under 4 years old must be secured in either a rear or forward-facing approved child restraint with an inbuilt harness.
- Children under 4 years old cannot travel in the front seat of a vehicle with two or more rows of seating.

---

2 www.choice.com.au/reviews-and-tests/babies-and-kids/travel/transport/child-car-restraints-review-and-compare.aspx

- Children aged from 4 years old but under 7 years old must be secured in a forward-facing approved child restraint with an inbuilt harness or an approved booster seat.
- Children aged from 4 years old but under 7 years old cannot travel in the front seat of a vehicle with two or more rows of seating, unless all other back seats are occupied by children younger than 7 years in an approved child restraint or booster seat.[3]

Problem:	**Dirty baby capsule**
What to use:	**(exterior) Cake of bathroom soap, water, cloth; or uniodised salt, bucket; oil of cloves, spray pack; (interior) washing machine**
How to apply:	To clean a baby capsule, wipe the exterior, including the handles, with a cake of bathroom soap and water. Alternatively, wipe with a cloth with 1 cup of uniodised salt mixed in a 9 litre bucket of water. Wipe over the edges with a cloth sprayed with ¼ teaspoon oil of cloves in a 1 litre spray pack of water. Babies often suck on the edges, and baby spit is a combination of milk and moisture – an ideal environment for mould to grow. Most capsule interiors have a lining that can be removed and washed in the washing machine. It's best to use liners made of cotton.

---

3 www.childcarseats.com.au/legal-requirements

How to include siblings

Many siblings feel left out when a new baby arrives, so involve them in activities such as:

- Playing, singing and reading to the baby.
- Helping with laundry – such as passing the pegs or folding the washing.
- When the baby is older, they can brush baby's hair – brushes are very soft.
- Make the sibling's bedtime special.

Unless they are 5 years or older, don't allow children to change a baby's nappy and then only do so on the floor. If changing a cloth nappy, don't let them use pins.

 If sewing items for your baby, wash the material first to remove the dressing, and make sure you work in a clean environment.

How to choose a cot

Your baby will be in a cot for up to 3 years. Check that:

- The cot is certified to the Australian safety standard.
- It has a strong drop side so the baby can't climb out. There have been several product failures relating to drop sides in cots supplied in the US. Testing in Australia has identified some slat disengagement from drop side rails from poorly applied adhesives or badly aligned and joined slats. Test the cot by grabbing and shaking the slats or filler bars to

see if they are loose or weak.[4] If faulty, return the cot to the retailer.

- It's stable – make sure the cot doesn't rock around.
- It has a safe slat width – wide enough that a toddler can't climb out or get hands or feet stuck but narrow enough that a baby's head can't get stuck between the slats.

Check the height from the top of the mattress to the top of the rail. The ACCC suggests you take a tape measure when shopping so you can check the size of gaps and openings. Here's a checklist:

- The mattress must fit snugly to within 20 mm of sides and ends.
- With the mattress base set in a fixed or lower position, the distance between the top of the mattress base and the top edge of the lowest cot side must be at least 600 mm when access is closed or 250 mm when access is open, or in an upper base position at least 400 mm when access is closed or 250 mm when access is open.
- The spacing between the bars or panels in the cot sides and ends needs to be between 50 mm and 95 mm – gaps wider than 95 mm can trap a child's head. If the bars or panels are made from flexible material, the maximum spacing between the bars or panels should be less than 95 mm.
- Check that there are no spaces between 30 mm and 50 mm that could trap your child's arms or legs.

---

4   www.productsafety.gov.au/content/index.phtml/itemId/980675

- Check that there are no small holes or openings between 5 mm and 12 mm wide that small fingers can be caught in.
- Check there are no fittings (including bolts, knobs and corner posts) that might catch onto your child's clothing and cause distress or strangulation.[5]

While we're talking about safety, be careful with second-hand and heirloom cots. As the ACCC warns, these can be a hazard to children because:

- The spacing between the bars may be too wide and trap a child's head, or may be too narrow and trap a child's arms or legs.
- The corner posts of the cot may be higher than the sides and ends, creating a strangulation hazard if clothes get caught on them.
- The catches on the side of the cot may be easy for a child to undo.
- Older cots may be painted with lead paint that children might chew on and swallow when they are teething.[6]

 TIP If you have an antique cot, test it with a lead safety kit. Check that catches are easy to undo – you can use baby-safe cupboard lockers. If there's any roughness, smooth it with sandpaper. If the item has value and you can't smooth it, cover hazardous areas or don't use the cot at all.

---

5 www.accc.gov.au/system/files/Cot%20safety%20-%20safety%20alert.pdf
6 www.accc.gov.au/system/files/Cot%20safety%20-%20safety%20alert.pdf

Highchairs

The highchair will be covered in your culinary creations. When choosing one, consider ease of cleaning, safety and durability. Here's a checklist:

- Look for a three-strap harness – the tray is not enough (the baby may slide underneath it).
- The wider the tray, the more food it will catch.
- Make sure the base is sturdy – the legs should be splayed 10 per cent wider than the top of the chair so it doesn't topple over.
- Make sure the locking mechanism is sturdy.
- Keep highchairs away from walls and other furniture so the child can't push the highchair over.
- Make sure the highchair is comfy to sit on with adequate padding or cushioning.

If you have a choice, opt for stitched vinyl rather than heat-fused vinyl seams because the latter can break more easily and expose the foam underneath.

The tray must be able to be locked into position or you could get bruised fingers. Make sure your baby's hands are clear of the tray when putting it into place. If you have an old highchair, screw a rubber stopper on the underside of the tray so it can't squash fingers.

Prams and strollers

Buying a pram or stroller is almost like buying a car: there are so many to choose from and they can cost a fortune. The most important factor is how practical it is. Make sure the pram or stroller:

- Is strong and stable.
- Is able to be opened and closed easily.
- Has good steering – a stroller with a bar across the top is easier to manage than one with two single handles.
- Has adjustable wheel action – look for locking actions on the wheels so you can manage different terrains and spaces, and check the brakes.
- Has comfy seating with a recline option and seat belts.
- Has good suspension – to make the journey smoother.
- Is able to face front or back – the handles should move front to back.
- Has a space for bags and other items underneath.

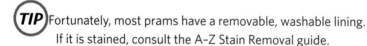 **TIP** Fortunately, most prams have a removable, washable lining. If it is stained, consult the A–Z Stain Removal guide.

How to choose a change table

The ideal height of a change table is to the height of your elbow when you are standing so you won't have to bend an already sore back. Choose a padded change table with a securing strap so the baby doesn't roll off.

Never leave a baby unattended on the change table – always have one hand on them, even if they're strapped in. Everything you need to change the baby should be within easy reach.

Have a disposal system, such as buckets for cloth nappies and bags with ties for disposable nappies. Choose bags that are environmentally friendly and lightly perfumed. Ensure that the surface of the change table can be sterilised. To test, add a single drop of water to the surface. If the water is absorbed, don't buy it. The length of the table should be 900 mm.

There is no Australian Standard for baby change tables. CHOICE tests for:

- stability
- strength of construction
- roll-off protection
- sharp edges and protrusions
- gaps or holes that could trap a small finger or limb (these are tested with a set of special probes).

CHAPTER 2

SLEEPING

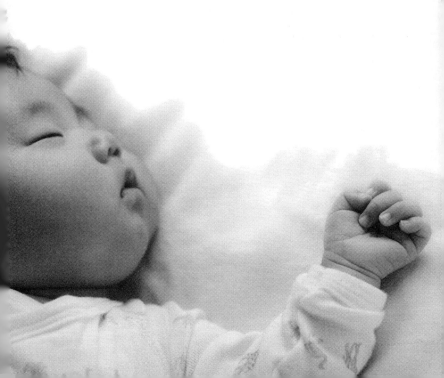

The amount your baby sleeps is a bit of a lottery. You could be blessed with a dream sleeper or your baby could wake every couple of hours. According to the experts, for the first 6 to 12 months, your baby should sleep in their own cot or bassinette in the same room as you.[7] Create a calm, hygienic space and avoid bright décor until they move to their own room.

7   www.sidsandkids.org/wp-content/uploads/SafeSleeping_Brochure.pdf

PREPARING THE BABY'S ROOM

The baby's room should be cool and airy, without extremes of heat and cold. Avoid strong perfumes or air fresheners because they can irritate your baby's lungs. And something you may not know: don't put flowers or potted plants in a room where a baby sleeps. Potting mixture contains dangerous microbes that travel easily. Air plants are safe.

Place the cot free standing rather than hard against a wall because the temperature of a wall changes and will affect the baby. Leave a full hand span around the cot on all sides. The most convenient position to locate a cot, if you can, is at the centre of the room because it's easier to access. If you're concerned about bed bugs, put each foot of the cot into a small bowl of water – bed bugs can't cross water. This will stop ants as well.

Each week, wash sheets and pillowcases in water hotter than 55°C. If washing in cold water, add a little eucalyptus oil or tea tree oil to the fabric conditioner slot of the washing machine to deal with dust mites.

Consider noise levels

Babies are very sensitive to sound and will easily startle. If sudden noises are common near the room, set up white noise, such as having a radio on low volume. If the floorboards are creaky, place a rug on the floor to reduce noise and disturbance when you check on your baby. To reduce echo in the room, place a small piece of rubber under the feet of the cot and under each piece of furniture. If you live on a busy road or have a barking dog next door, cut bubble wrap to the size of the window with the bubble side fixed to the glass. Attach with a removable adhesive. Cover all windows in the room to create a baffle. Soft furnishings, such as a big chair, will also absorb sound.

Another noisy item to consider is baby monitors. Make sure they don't burp and beep because this will wake the baby.

 If you are using a baby monitor, be sure to follow the instructions carefully. If the monitor isn't set up correctly and the cord is pulled into the cot, it may become wrapped around a child's neck and pose a risk of strangulation. If your baby monitor has cords attached, ensure the cords are inaccessible to a baby or child.

Check for draughts

To find draughts, light a candle and walk around the room watching the flicker of the flame. If the flame bends, it indicates a draught. Check areas where air can get in – such as doors, floors (especially floorboards) and skirting boards. To fix draughts, cover the access area, place a mat over the floor or use self-adhesive tape to cover gaps.

⚠ WARNING
Don't hang mobiles across or above cots.
Mobiles can be dangerous and over-stimulating for babies. The cot is a place for sleeping, not playing. Place mobiles near change tables.

TIP Keep a comfy chair in the baby's room for feeding and snoozing. If you have a specific feeding spot, it helps with your baby's sleep routine. Rocking chairs are ideal, with some especially designed for baby feeding and rocking.

TIP Babies love nursery rhymes, especially when you sing to them. Plenty of recordings and lyrics (in case you've forgotten the words) are available online.

⚠ WARNING
Check for cords.
Never have dangly items, including cords from blinds, within reach of the cot or the baby could become entangled. Consider what the baby will be able to reach and whether it's safe.

Modern heaters have an auto-off switch in case they are tipped over, but still be careful using them. Make sure there are no flammable items nearby and never have an electric bar heater where a child can reach it. Install a smoke alarm in the baby's room, just in case.

SIDS guidelines[8]

SIDS (or Sudden Infant Death Syndrome) is when a baby dies suddenly, without warning, while they are asleep. For more information visit www.sidsandkids.org. Safe sleeping practices include:

- Sleep baby on their back from birth – never on the tummy or side.
- Sleep baby with head and face uncovered.
- Avoid exposing babies to cigarette smoke, before and after birth.
- Provide a safe sleeping environment, night and day: safe cot, safe mattress, safe bedding and safe sleeping place.
- Sleep baby in their own cot or bassinette in the same room as the parents for the first 6 to 12 months.

To provide a safe sleeping environment for your baby:
- Put baby's feet at the bottom of the cot.
- The cot must meet Australian standards.
- No additional mattresses or extra padding should be placed in a travel cot.

---

8 www.sidsandkids.org/wp-content/uploads/SafeSleeping_Brochure.pdf

- Tuck in bedclothes securely so bedding is not loose.
- Keep quilts, doonas, duvets, pillows, cot bumpers, sheepskins and soft toys out of the cot or sleeping place.
- Use a firm, clean mattress that fits snugly in the cot.
- Bean bags of any kind should never be used for a baby to sleep or nap in as they could cause suffocation.

 TIP Wipe lavender oil around door and window frames to freshen the room and assist with sleeping.

Remove toys from cots

If your baby is under 7 months of age, don't keep soft toys in the cot because the toy could cover the baby's nose and mouth and interfere with breathing. According to SIDS and Kids WA, 'Small toys, toy parts and toys on strings are a major cause of asphyxial fatalities caused by accidental suffocation and strangulation in babies and choking episodes in young children. Toys which are hung across the cot should be removed once the child can push on hands and knees or is 5 months of age; whichever comes earliest.'[9]

Some toys are scented with talcum powder but this is dangerous for babies because it could restrict their breathing. After 7 months, only allow toys or comforters in the cot that are made of terry towelling or materials that a child can breathe through as they sleep.

---

9 www.sidsandkidswa.org/assets/info-statements/soft-toys-in-the-cot-_2013-mar-final1[1].pdf

DID YOU KNOW? If you are concerned about the safety of your child's cot or other items, check the Australian Competition and Consumer Commission's product recalls list online at www.recalls.gov.au. At the time of writing, several cots had been recalled because of failures with labelling, drop sides, dimensions, sharp edges and points, and marking requirements.

Baby mattress

Shannon prefers a tea tree mattress for babies up to 6 months old because it allows good airflow around the baby and inhibits insects.

After 6 months, the baby is too heavy for the tea tree and you'll need a foam or inner spring mattress. Make sure the mattress fits the cot properly – you shouldn't be able to fit more than two fingers (20 mm) between the mattress and the edge of the cot. The mattress should be quite firm. If you are concerned about gassing in mattresses, organic mattresses are available.

Whatever the type of mattress, use a mattress protector because there are bound to be spills and leaks and it's much easier to clean a mattress protector than a mattress. Choose one that is washable and breathable, and that secures underneath the mattress. Don't use those with elastic bands on each corner – these are a potential hazard. Most mattress protectors have a terry towelling top and plasticised surface underneath. Wash when wet; don't leave urine, vomit or spills to dry.

Sheets and bedding

Sheets and blankets should always be well tucked so the baby can't unwrap them and become tangled. Shannon's mum taught her to fit an adult-sized sheet for the base sheet. Fit it diagonally and fold underneath the mattress like an envelope. Avoid elasticised or fitted sheets because they can become loose. Use only 100 per cent cotton sheets – never nylon or polyester. When nylon or polyester gets wet, it creates a moisture barrier and could cause a rash. Synthetic fibres also hold smells and are harder to keep hygienic.

Cover the baby with light cotton blankets, cotton bunny rugs or cotton waffle blankets. Tuck blankets in short-sheeted so the baby can't wrap a blanket over their head. Blankets should sit at the line of the baby's shoulder. This ensures that if they get under the blanket, they can't seal it over themselves.

As a rule, babies don't need pillows or cot bumpers – it's safer not to use a pillow until they are 2 years old.

A baby's bed should be aired every day. This means stripping the sheets and blankets from the mattress and hanging them over the edge of the cot. This is important because babies are susceptible to bacteria and infection. Babies don't sweat as easily as adults and have more dead skin cells, so wash sheets every 3 days or when wet. If any bedding is wet, wash it straightaway. If the bedding is urine stained, remove the stain as soon as possible.

Cleaning routine

Harsh chemical cleaners, such as bleach, are far more toxic
and harmful than dirt. Instead, clean your baby's room with
good old soap and water. Every day, wipe over the cot with a
damp, soapy cloth; babies suck on the bars. Wipe over hard
surfaces with a cloth sprayed with ¼ teaspoon of tea tree oil in
1 litre of water, or 1 teaspoon of lavender oil in 1 litre of water,
mixed in a spray bottle. Have one cloth covered with spray and
another dry cloth. Wipe the cot with one, before drying with
the other. If you have a mosquito net, wash it when washing
the sheets. Clean a toddler's room twice a week. Vacuum
regularly because children are susceptible to dust and dust
mites.

Problem:	**Urine stain on mattress**
What to use:	**White vinegar or dishwashing liquid, cold water, cloth or old toothbrush, sunshine or hair dryer, lemon juice**
How to apply:	Tightly wring a cloth in white vinegar so it's damp but not wet. Blot over the stain. Alternatively, add a little dishwashing liquid to cold water to generate a sudsy mix. Scrub only the suds into the stain with a cloth or old toothbrush. In both cases, put the mattress in the sun. If this isn't possible, absorb moisture with paper towel (with a book on top) and dry with a hair dryer. Neutralise the urine smell by wiping with lemon juice on a cloth.

Problem: **Poo stain on mattress**

What to use: **Plastic comb or paper towel, cake of bathroom soap, cold water, cloth, dishwashing liquid, sunshine or hair dryer**

How to apply: Remove excess by lifting with a plastic comb or by blotting with paper towel. Scribble with a cake of bathroom soap run under cold water. Wipe with a damp cloth. Massage with a couple of drops of dishwashing liquid on your fingertips until the liquid feels like jelly. Wipe with a damp cloth until the dishwashing liquid is removed. Absorb moisture by covering the area with paper towel. If you can, place the mattress in sunshine. If not, dry using a hair dryer.

Vomit in cot

Q: 'My baby vomited in her cot. It went all over the sheets and all through the mattress,' reports Kate. 'She only drinks milk and eats vegetables but it's incredible how much mess a small baby can produce. I've already scrubbed the surface of the mattress and it still smells. What can I do?'

Problem: **Baby vomit in mattress**

What to use: **Washing machine, plastic comb or paper towel, cloth, lemon juice, water, spray pack, sunshine or hair dryer**

How to apply: Wash sheets in the washing machine on the cold setting. Remove excess vomit from the mattress by lifting with a plastic comb or by blotting with paper towel. Wipe with a damp cloth. To get rid of the smell, mix 1 tablespoon of lemon juice with 1 litre of

Cleaning nose syringes, nasal pumps and vaporisers

If your baby's nostrils are blocked, gently clear them with a baby nose syringe or nasal pump. Sterilise these in the same way as bottles – in hot, salted water. If your baby has the sniffles, an old-fashioned remedy is to express a little breast milk into a cup, draw a small amount into a syringe and gently squirt it into one of your baby's nostrils. It will make your baby sneeze and help clear congestion.

Avoid using vaporisers unless recommended by your doctor, and never add menthols – just use water. To clean vaporisers, mix 2 tablespoons of bicarb, 2 tablespoons of white vinegar and 2 tablespoons of uncooked rice. Place inside the vaporiser, shake and rinse with cold water.

If you use a vaporiser in a bedroom, it will become damp and mouldy. For this reason, it's better to use a vaporiser in the bathroom. Stay with your baby during the process. Clean the vaporiser every time you use it. Rinse with warm water and make sure it's completely dry before returning it to the cupboard.

water in a spray pack and spray over the
mattress. If you can, put the mattress in
the sun to dry it out and to kill bacteria.
Otherwise, dry with a hair dryer.

Sheepskin

Skeepskin in a cot is a SIDS risk because soft surfaces
are more likely to result in bub's face being covered, which
will affect their breathing. Once your baby can roll or sit up,
you can use sheepskins inside prams or on the floor during
play.

Swaddling wraps

Many newborns like to be wrapped as they sleep and there
are many swaddling wraps to choose from. As you'd expect,
natural fibres are best. Muslin is very common but can be
difficult to secure. Other options include fitted wraps made
with stretch cotton. You can also make your own swaddling
wrap. When buying cotton gauze from the fabric store, the
width and length should be the same, so you can create a
square. Buy 100 per cent cotton gauze and cut it to size, then
stitch the edging. You can wash the wrap in the washing
machine with the baby's clothing. A wrap is also handy to
throw over the carrier or pram to keep bugs out – it's light
enough for your baby to breathe through. Make sure you don't
wrap your baby too tightly.

How to wrap your baby

- Spread out a lightweight cotton or muslin wrap and fold the top over by 20 cm. Lay baby on the wrap with their shoulders in line with the fold. Place one of baby's hands under the fold.
- Bring the edge of the wrap across the body. Tuck it under baby's legs. Place their other hand under the fold.
- Bring the other edge of the wrap across baby's body. Tuck it in under the baby's back.
- Fold any extra length up and under baby's legs.

Graphite powder spill

Q: 'My husband was lubricating the baby's bedroom door hinges with graphite powder and spilt it over the sisal wool-blend carpet in that corner of the room,' says Simone. 'I have tried vacuuming it up but with no luck. Any suggestions?'

Problem:	**Graphite powder on carpet**
What to use:	**Cake of bathroom soap, cold water, damp cloth, paper towel**
How to apply:	Graphite and other fine powders are often left behind after vacuuming. To pick up fine matter, dampen a cake of bathroom soap with cold water and dab it up and down

over the graphite spots on the carpet. The graphite will stick to the soap. For a large spill, keep a bucket of cold water next to you and dip as you go. Remove excess soap with a damp cloth. Apply paper towel to remove moisture. Alternatively, cut the soap into a sausage shape by cutting lengthways and trimming the corners with a warm knife. Roll the soap backwards and forwards over the carpet.

(To prevent this problem, lubricate hinges with sewing machine oil or baby oil. Put newspaper or some other covering underneath the door when applying graphite powder or anything that can spill.)

Mosquito nettings for cots

Because babies are sensitive, they can react quite severely to insect bites. One way to protect them from mozzies is to place a mosquito net over the cot. Ensure the netting is large enough to cover the entire cot and that the bottom sits below the rungs so the baby can't pull the netting into the cot. Some netting has an elastic hem to hold it in place, or you can secure it by placing elastic over the top of the mosquito netting, like a garter, so there are no gaps for mozzies and other bugs to get in. Wash the netting regularly and hang in sunshine to dry. Add 2 drops of lavender oil to the rinse water in the washing machine to deter mozzies.

Deter mosquitoes by adding 2 drops of lavender oil to a 250 ml bottle of baby oil and use this mixture to massage the baby's skin. Never apply lavender oil directly to the skin because it's very concentrated. This applies to all essential oils.

Dummies/pacifiers checklist

The ACCC recommends that you:

- Check dummies before each use. Pull firmly on the teat and tug the handle and ring to ensure they don't give way under pressure.
- Check the teat for wear and tear. If it looks worn or damaged, throw the dummy away.
- Store dummies away from direct sunlight, which can cause the rubber or silicone to perish.
- Sterilise dummies or wash them in hot soapy water; then rinse in boiled water and air dry.
- Regularly buy new dummies, as constant use and washing causes them to weaken.

Watch children who can remove dummies themselves because they're more likely to place the entire dummy into their mouth, not just the teat.

Ditch the dummy

Breaking the dummy habit can be hard. Here are some suggestions:

- The Gradual Phase-out – scale back dummy use to bedtime only and substitute with a bottle.
- The Sabotage – cut the tip off the rubber teat so it doesn't suction as well.
- The Fantasy Story – tell them Santa needs the dummies for the baby reindeers and will come to collect them. Or tell them the 'dummy fairy' is coming.
- The Self Phase-out – wait for them to outgrow the dummy.

Bassinette basics

Bassinettes are only suitable until 3 months of age or when your baby's weight reaches 9 kilos, whichever comes first. When selecting a bassinette, follow these guidelines from the ACCC:

- A wide, stable base so the bassinette won't tip over.
- A size and style to suit your baby's weight and age.
- Sides at least 300 mm higher than the top of the mattress base, to stop your baby from falling out.
- A firm, snug-fitting mattress – no more than 75 mm thick – to prevent suffocation.
- If the legs fold, ensure they can be locked and won't collapse when used.
- Short decorative trims and bows that can't strangle your baby – or better still, a bassinette without decorative trims. Long decorations could cause strangulation.

Clean in the same way as a cot – with a damp, soapy cloth. Wash the lining in the washing machine and dry in sunshine.

How to clean a baby bouncer or bouncinette

Baby bouncers are suitable for babies until 9 months. Because they don't have any traction, always watch your baby in a bouncer in case it topples. Avoid feeding your baby in a bouncer because food and crumbs go everywhere, necessitating extra cleaning. Baby bouncers are great for settling babies – pump the base with your foot to create a rocking motion. Be aware that bouncinettes, prams and strollers are not designed for a baby to sleep in. If your baby does fall asleep in one, they must be supervised. When you can, transfer them to their cot or bed.

Problem:	**Dirty covering on baby bouncer/ bouncinette**
What to use:	**Washing machine, sunshine**
How to apply:	Remove the cotton covering and wash it in the washing machine. Dry it in sunshine.

 TIP Turn a double bed into a temporary baby safe sleeping zone by placing pillows around the edge of the bed and spreading a blanket over the top of the bed and pillows. The weight of the baby on the blanket holds the pillows in place.

Moving from a cot to a bed

When your child can climb out of a cot, it's time for a bed. Kids' beds should be firm with a soft top. The firm base keeps their spines straight and the soft top stops them from feeling sore on pressure points. Create a soft top by placing a 1 cm thick sheet of foam rubber over the mattress or use a sheepskin covering. Because both are washable, they are ideal for children who have allergies.

What to do about bed-wetters

One in three 4-year-olds wets the bed – it's much more common that you'd expect. One reason could be that the bladder isn't fully formed, particularly in boys. Don't harass a child who wets the bed. The most successful treatment is a bedwetting alarm that can be hired. Ask your GP about these. Other suggestions include:

- Take your child for a walk half an hour before bedtime so fluid is pushed through their kidneys more quickly.
- Don't let your child have a drink before sleeping.
- Put plastic underneath the sheets.
- If there are continuing problems, seek medical advice.

Greasy nightie

Q: 'My daughter was given a new nightie by her nanna,' says Patrick, 'but I'd been washing grease off my truck and it ended up on the nightie. Needless to say, I'm not too popular. Can the nightie be fixed?'

Problem: **Truck grease on fabric**
What to use: **Baby oil, dishwashing liquid**
How to apply: This is a difficult job. First, rub the grease spots with baby oil to dilute the stain. Then rub over the spots with a couple of drops of dishwashing liquid on your fingers. Rinse under blood-heat (body temperature) water. Wash in the washing machine. It may be easier to buy a new nightie.

CHAPTER 3

FEEDING

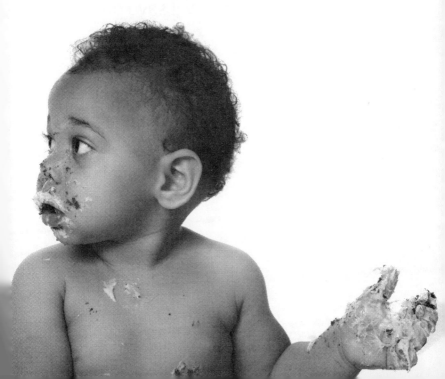

Once you get into a routine, feeding is a wonderful time to connect with your baby. When they grow into a toddler, meal times can become a challenge, with food going everywhere but their mouth. Fortunately, most trays, tables and other eating surfaces are easy to clean and the right bib will save on cleaning.

FEEDING BABY

While not every mother is able to breastfeed, there are many benefits from doing so, not only for bub but for mum, too. Breastfeeding helps to rebalance hormones and get your body back into shape after birth. And it's much more convenient than sterilising bottles and preparing formula. Your baby's brain also benefits by engaging in a positive sensory exchange with you as they feed. In Australia, it's recommended that infants be exclusively breastfed until around 6 months of age, when solid foods are introduced. Breastfeeding can continue until 12 months and beyond, if the mother and child want to.[10] If you can, 'breast is best'. But don't worry if you can't breastfeed. According to an article in *Scientific American*, rather than just the contents of your milk, it's the experience of being in mum's or dad's arms and making a connection as your baby feeds from the bottle that counts.[11]

Whether you breastfeed or bottle feed, you're bound to have some spills and stains. Prevention is always best, so when feeding, keep a damp cloth handy to wipe away any spills when they happen. This is much easier than dealing with a stain later on. In the first 6 months, the most common spill will be breast milk or formula; both are high in proteins, so remove using cold water – hot water sets protein stains.

---

10 www.nhmrc.gov.au/_files_nhmrc/publications/attachments/n56b_infant_feeding_summary_130808.pdf

11 www.scientificamerican.com/article/surety-bond-breast-feeding/

Problem:	**Spit-up breast milk or formula**
What to use:	**Cake of bathroom soap, cold water, stiff brush**
How to apply:	It's common for babies to spit-up partially digested milk, particularly if they have reflux. This spit-up milk contains gastric juices including hydrochloric acid. To clean spit-up stains, scribble with a cake of bathroom soap and cold water. Formula is more difficult to remove, so scrub over the soap with a stiff brush. To prevent these stains when feeding, put a rubber-backed towel or cloth over your shoulder to catch the spit-up. This will also rescue your clothes from the lamington look caused by the unavoidable pale fluff from baby clothes. Shannon's solution: hide baby spit-up stains by wearing light-coloured clothes.

When feeding, have a comfortable chair to sit on. Choose one with arms, so you can rest your elbows against them and support the baby's head. To relieve pressure on your arm, place a pillow underneath your arm in line with the baby's spine. Place the chair in a quiet, comfortable area. The calmer you and your baby are while feeding, the less likely the baby will get gas and stomach cramps. If you're comfortable, your milk will flow more easily, too.

TIP Keep a safety pin on your bra strap to remind you what side you're up to when feeding. Swap the pin right or left with each feed.

If you have issues feeding, lactation specialists can offer advice and assistance. Ask for a recommendation at your local early childhood health centre. These centres also offer regular appointments and baby check-ups, parenting courses, baby feeding help, childhood immunisation clinics and specialist services. The **healthdirect Australia pregnancy, birth & baby line (1800 882 436)** offers advice 24 hours a day. There's information on feeding in the National Health and Medical Research Council infant feeding guidelines.[12]

BABY BOTTLES

Baby bottles come in many shapes, materials and sizes; common sizes are 120 ml and 225 ml. Many have 'venting technology' to prevent air bubbles from being ingested by your baby. Glass bottles are popular again because of concerns about some of the chemicals used to make plastics. Glass is more expensive than plastic but lasts longer, and you can buy protective silicone coverings. If you use plastic bottles, discard them if they become scratched or cloudy; it means the plastic has degraded, and bacteria can penetrate. If you breastfeed but occasionally use a bottle, choose a teat with a wide-based nipple like a breast. Some babies find it difficult to switch

---

12 www.nhmrc.gov.au/guidelines/publications/n56

from breast to teat if there's a big difference in shape and size. Bottle-fed babies don't have this issue. Teats are made of silicone, latex or rubber – silicone is more durable but the choice will depend on what your baby prefers.

DID YOU KNOW? Breast milk digests more easily than formula, so a breastfed baby gets hungry more often.

Should you avoid polycarbonate baby bottles?

Before 2011, many plastic baby bottles contained Bisphenol A (BPA) to make them clear and shatterproof. But a few years ago, there were concerns that tiny amounts of BPA could leach from the plastic into milk. In 2010, Food Standards Australia New Zealand (FSANZ) evaluated the safety of BPA and plasticisers in polycarbonate baby bottles and concluded that levels of BPA or plasticisers were very low and did not pose a risk to babies' health. Even so, most of Australia's big retailers phased out the sale of baby bottles containing BPA. This followed bans on the use of BPA in baby bottles in Europe and the United States.

A 2010 study commissioned by the Australian Consumer and Competition Commission found that:

Typical infant feeding bottles and infant sip cups that are currently available on the Australian market do not expose infants to detectable amounts of Bisphenol A and are safe for their intended purpose. In terms of potential infant exposure to Bisphenol A, there is no discernable difference in safety between the use of glass, non-polycarbonate plastic and polycarbonate plastic infant feeding vessels.[13]

In the case of exposure from other sources of BPA, such as canned goods, FSANZ cites a survey undertaken by CHOICE that found that:

a nine month old baby weighing 9 kg would have to eat more than 1 kg of canned baby custard containing BPA every day to reach the TDI (Tolerable Daily Intake), assuming that the custard contained the highest level of BPA found (420 parts per billion).[14]

If you have plastic bottles containing BPA, use cold sterilising product and rinse thoroughly. To work out if a bottle contains BPA, look at the injection joins. BPA is slightly different in colour. Don't heat these bottles in a microwave. Instead, place milk inside and warm the bottle in a bowl of hot water.

 The times of day at which you eat while pregnant will become the most active times for your baby once it is born. You may want to change your eating times during pregnancy to encourage earlier mealtimes for your baby.

---

13 www.productsafety.gov.au/content/item.phtml?itemId=982022&nodeId=64e
999914413550d78f07f9c93a789e0&fn=BPA%20in%20Bottles%20-%20Test%20
Report.pdf

14 www.foodstandards.gov.au/consumer/chemicals/bpa/Pages/default.aspx

How to clean and sterilise bottles and teats

Until your baby is at least 6 months old, ensure you clean and sterilise their feeding equipment. Baby immune systems are still developing and hygiene is paramount. And don't allow other children to use their feeding equipment.

To clean

- Breast milk and formula are both high in proteins and sugars. Rinse bottles with cold water first until no milk remains (hot water sets proteins). Rinse bottles as soon after feeding as possible.
- After rinsing, wash bottles in the sink in warm water and a little dishwashing liquid. Use a bottle brush to clean the inside of bottles.
- Rinse in clean water, then sterilise.

To sterilise

- Fill a large pot with water and add 2 tablespoons of salt. Bring to the boil.
- Place bottles and teats inside.
- Turn off the heat and leave for 10 minutes.
- Rinse the bottles in boiled water (hot or cold) to remove residual salt. Allow to air dry.

If you can, avoid using the dishwasher to clean bottles and teats (and anything that comes into contact with baby's mouth) because of detergent residue. If you must use a dishwasher, rinse bottles with cold water first, and rinse them again in boiling water after they come out of the dishwasher.

Once your baby is over 6 months, you can use the dishwasher, but replace the detergent with bicarb and white vinegar. Use the same amount of bicarb as you would detergent in the detergent dispenser. Add white vinegar rather than rinse-aid product to the rinse dispenser. If washing other dishes at the same time, you will still need to rinse the bottles after washing.

 Store boiled water in a sterile container in the fridge. It will come in handy.

Commercial sterilising products are available, but Shannon doesn't think they are necessary. Salt and boiling water work perfectly well. Don't stack baby bottles alongside your regular household washing; dish racks are often dirty. You can buy dish racks especially designed for baby bottles. After rinsing, cover the bottles with a clean tea towel.

How to sterilise utensils

Any item that goes into a baby's mouth should be sterilised. This includes bottles, dummies or pacifiers, teats, spoons, medication pipettes or syringes, sippy cups and gum massagers. Store baby utensils separately (a container with a lid is ideal) to keep them sterile. Keep a couple of spare dummies, as they're often dropped on the ground.

Avoid the temptation to stick a dropped dummy back in your baby's mouth. You sucking the dropped dummy before putting it in their mouth doesn't count – saliva doesn't sterilise.

Problem: Dirty utensils

What to use: Pot, salt, water

How to apply: Place 2 tablespoons of salt in a pot of water, bring to the boil, turn the heat off, add items and leave for 10 minutes. Then rinse with boiled water.

⚠ WARNING

Don't let other people put their fingers in your baby's mouth. It's one of the most common ways for a baby to get oral thrush.

Put on the bib

Bibs are a perfect way to protect baby clothing from stains during feeding, although sometimes they don't catch everything. Most are made from plastic or cotton, often with plastic backing; some have pockets to catch food. When self-feeding begins, some bibs aren't big enough and don't protect clothing.

Cleaning bibs

To clean cotton bibs

- Soak immediately after feeding – dried stains are always more difficult to remove.
- After washing, hang in the sunshine. The UV in sunlight fades stains.
- Keep several bibs on-hand and ready to use.

To clean bibs with plastic backing

- Wash immediately after use or they go mouldy very quickly. Saliva is ideal incubation for mould.

To clean plastic/rubber bibs

- Scrape food into the bin or compost bucket.
- Wipe bib with a damp cloth or rinse under water.

 If your baby has cracks around their nostrils, apply papaw cream. Ears can also become cracked – use papaw or another suitable lotion. Any cream or lotion your baby can touch with their hands needs to be orally safe. If unsafe, make it inaccessible to little hands.

Yellow bottles and teats

Q: 'All the bottles and teats we use have developed a yellowish tinge. I wash the bottles in soapy water (both hot and cold sterilising). Can I make them clear again?' asks Belinda.

Problem:	**Yellowish tinge on bottles and teats**
What to use:	**Large pot, salt, water**
How to apply:	The yellow tinge means the plastic is burnt, probably from using commercial sterilisation products that contain chlorine. To prevent this, after rinsing bottles and teats, fill a large pot with water and add 2 tablespoons of salt. Bring to the boil. Place bottles and

teats inside. Turn off the heat and leave for 10 minutes. Rinse the bottles in boiled water (hot or cold) to remove residual salt. Allow to air dry. If yellowing remains, throw out the bottles because they are unsafe to use.

Baby medicines

Most baby medicines contain sugar-like substances that are sticky and need to be rinsed off clothing with warm water. Dry in sunshine if you can. Droppers need to be rinsed with warm water and then sterilised. Keep medicines out of reach of children, not only for safety but to avoid spillage.

DID YOU KNOW? After giving birth, your mood can be affected because hormones need time to rebalance and protein is drained from your body to create milk for the baby. You may want to try these remedies.
- Drink camomile tea – a great relaxant.
- Eat plenty of fresh fruit, vegetables and protein.
- Drink fennel tea – this helps with milk production. In the first month, you'll experience up and down days. On a down day, the baby gets stressed and you get stressed. A cup of fennel tea will speed your milk delivery and ease the baby's stomach.

Should you use antibacterial hand sanitisers and wipes?

Good hygiene is important, but there's no need for 'germ panic'. Even though many antibacterial hand sanitisers are available, according to Trent Yarwood, Infectious Diseases Physician and lecturer at the University of Queensland:

> We do not – and cannot – live in a germ-free world. Spending money on these products doesn't guarantee you won't get sick (of course they can't) and they probably don't even *reduce* your risk of getting sick. But they might contribute to bacterial resistance, and they certainly cost more. Break the marketing cycle of germ panic and reach for the plain old soap.[15]

Practise good food-handling techniques and wash your hands.

To minimise the volume of bacteria, don't cut up meat on the same chopping board as vegetables without washing the board before each use. Children should never be exposed to uncooked meat. Wash vegetables and fruit in a bowl with a small amount of salt water.

DID YOU KNOW? When you breastfeed, your baby reacts to the food you eat. Until your baby is around 4 months old, you eating strawberries could cause them to break out in a rash. When you reintroduce foods, after feeding your baby wait for 24 hours before consuming the food again and watch if there's a reaction. If there's a rash, omit the food and try again a month later.

---

15 http://theconversation.com/health-check-should-i-use-antibacterial-hand-sanitisers-21384

Other things to keep in mind about your own diet:

- Unpeeled fruit should be washed before eating because it's often covered in wax. This isn't a problem for adults, but could cause a reaction in babies through breast milk.
- Garlic and onions in large quantities can cause gas in babies.
- Ask your baby health clinic or doctor about eating nuts because there's conflicting information. Recent research suggests allergies could be related to particular gut microbes.[16]

 If your baby is constipated, consult your family doctor or baby health clinic. You might have to change formula or, if your baby is over 6 months, increase their intake of fruit and vegetables or give them diluted prune juice. An old-fashioned remedy is to mix ¼ teaspoon of brown sugar and ½ teaspoon of freshly squeezed orange juice in a bottle of boiled water. Give them additional boiled water for a couple of days.

Problem:	**Breast milk on carpet**
What to use:	**Paper towel, cake of bathroom soap, cold water, cloth**
How to apply:	Remove excess by blotting with paper towel. Scribble with a cake of bathroom soap run under cold water. Wipe with a damp cloth.

---

16 http://news.sciencemag.org/biology/2014/08/gut-microbe-stops-food-allergies?utm_source=nextdraft&utm_medium=email

Problem: **Baby formula on carpet**
What to use: **Paper towel, cake of bathroom soap,**
cold water, toothbrush, glycerine, cloth
How to apply: Baby formula is more difficult than breast
milk to remove because it contains artificially
created enzymes that bond to fats more easily.
Remove excess by blotting with paper towel.
Scribble with a cake of bathroom soap run
under cold water. Scrub with a toothbrush in
every direction – north, south, east and west.
If the stain is older than 1 hour, wipe with
2 drops of glycerine on a toothbrush in every
direction. Leave for 90 minutes. Then scribble
with a cake of bathroom soap. Wipe with a
damp cloth.

Problem: **Breast milk on wool**
What to use: **Cake of bathroom soap, cheap shampoo**
How to apply: Scribble with a cake of bathroom soap dipped
in cold water. Gently rub the wool against
itself using your hands. Wash straightaway in
1 teaspoon of cheap shampoo and blood-heat
(body temperature) water. Rinse in blood-heat
water. Gently wring and dry flat on a towel in
the shade.

TIP If reheating food in the microwave, avoid using plastic
containers. Instead, reheat food in ceramic, glass or
silicone containers.

Each time you prepare vegetables for yourself, cook extra, purée, place in an iceblock container and freeze. Once frozen, transfer cubes to a zip-lock bag, glass or silicone container and return to the freezer, ready to use instead of tinned baby food.

 Until the age of 10, simple foods are easier for children to digest. Reduce excess salt and sugars.

HIGHCHAIRS

The Australian Competition and Consumer Commission has this advice on highchair safety:

- Always use the harness or restraint system.
- Make sure your baby's hands are not in the way when you raise or lower the tray.
- Always watch your baby in the highchair and take your baby with you if you need to leave the room. Never leave your baby unsupervised.
- Stop your baby from standing or trying to climb out of or into the highchair.
- Position the highchair at least 500 mm away from windows, doors, stoves, electrical appliances and curtain or blind cords.
- Place the highchair out of your baby's reach when not in use.
- Check for loose or broken parts and exposed foam on the seat that could choke your baby.
- Never allow other children to play near or climb onto the highchair.

How to clean a highchair

To clean, wipe with a cake of bathroom soap and cold water on a damp cloth or pantyhose. For hardened food, place a damp cloth over the area and leave for 10 minutes. The food will come away when you wipe it down. To prevent mould, wipe with ¼ teaspoon oil of cloves in 1 litre of water in a spray pack applied with a cloth. Repeat once a month. If your child is messy, place a flat garbage bag under the highchair to catch food. Secure your baby in the highchair with a soft seat cover.

HOW TO MAKE A SOFT SEAT COVER

Buy cotton quilt fabric and cut it into a rectangle 30 cm x 20 cm in size. Make a cut in the middle of the shorter end on one side for the legs. At the other end, sew a long strap of the quilting fabric and attach Velcro to either end. The strap wraps around the baby and across the front of the highchair/trolley/pram. The Velcro means you can use it anywhere. Wash in the washing machine.

 TIP When feeding, only wipe your baby's face at the end of the meal, rather than throughout, to avoid their sensitive skin becoming chafed.

Baby spew on upholstery

Q: 'A recent visitor was breastfeeding her baby on my jacquard chair and the baby regurgitated milk on it,' says Karen. 'It has a dark stain that I can't seem to get out. What do you suggest?'

Problem:	**Baby vomit on upholstery**
What to use:	**Cake of bathroom soap, cloth, paper towel, unprocessed wheat bran, white vinegar, pantyhose**
How to apply:	If the stain has a dark edging, it's a protein stain. To remove, scribble with a cake of bathroom soap dipped in cold water and wipe with a damp cloth. Press with paper towel to absorb moisture. If there's a watermark, place 1 cup of unprocessed wheat bran in a large bowl. Add drops of white vinegar one at a time, stirring as you go, until the mixture resembles breadcrumbs. It shouldn't be wet. Place the mixture into the toe of the pantyhose and tie off tightly. It will be the size of a tennis ball. Rub over the stain until removed.

How to clean breast pumps

Clean any part of the pump that comes into contact with breast milk. You don't need to clean tubing unless it comes into contact with breast milk. First, rinse off any milk under cold water. Then boil a pot of water, turn off the heat, place any immersible items into the water and leave for 10 minutes. Rinse with boiled water. Allow tubing to air dry before reattaching to your breast pump. Wipe over hard parts with a damp cloth.

How to clean drinking and sippy cups

These can be a challenge to clean because they are designed to reduce spills and stains. In a sink of warm water, rinse the cup using a bottle brush (dedicated for this use). To clean rubber and bendy plastic, place a little salt on a clean toothbrush (have a dedicated one) and scrub. Rinse with water and the salt will dissolve. Sterilise the toothbrush as you would a baby bottle. After cleaning, store items in a sealed plastic container to protect from bacteria.

 Banana skin contains resins that can irritate a baby's skin, so only allow them to hold the flesh of a banana.

Introducing solids

Your baby health clinic consultant or doctor can tell you the ideal proportions of protein, vegetables, fat and carbohydrates to include in your baby or toddler's diet, which will change as they grow older. If you can, make baby food yourself so you know exactly what's in it. If you can't make your own baby food, test different commercial products until you find one that offers the best nutrition. Read the labels and don't use foods that have additives.

When your baby begins to eat solids, select a dedicated spot to place the highchair and reinforce the good habit of eating at the same spot each mealtime. Don't allow children to wander around the house when they eat. It can be dangerous. To prevent choking, make sure food is mashed and placed at the front of the mouth when eating. This makes children use their tongue and jaws to chew. You might have more dribble and spit, but that's easily sorted. If food is placed at the back of the mouth, they may not chew it properly.

Step by step to solid foods

This is how Shannon introduced solids to her children:

- Start with rice cereal because it's easiest to digest. Mix ½ teaspoon of rice cereal powder in 2 tablespoons of warm breast milk or formula. As they get used to textures, increase the proportion of rice cereal.

- Then introduce breads, such as rusks made of arrowroot. Start with a little of this sort of food and increase.

- Add fruit-based oils (such as olive oil) and seed-based oils (such as sunflower, canola and sesame oil), but not legume-based oils, which can contain nuts and cause an allergic reaction. Use butter rather than margarine because margarine contains legume-based oils.

- Add dairy foods (no cow's milk until 12 months) and simple fruits such as apple or pear. Some babies are lactose intolerant, so introduce dairy foods slowly. If your baby is intolerant, try goat's milk. Peel, slice and cook fruit until soft, then purée. Make four or five servings and freeze excess in an ice cube tray.

- Add vegetables – starch-based, including potato, sweet potato, pumpkin, carrot and yams. Cook and purée. Don't add salt.

- Add broccoli and spinach. When teeth come through, add lettuce and celery (one of the last vegetables to introduce your baby to, because it's fibrous).

- Add fish (not shellfish), meat, eggs and legumes. When introducing meat, give your baby a bone to suck on – especially when they're teething. Don't feed them meals with multiple ingredients until 9 months.
- Add stone fruits last because they are high in sulphur, which can cause diarrhoea.

 TIP When your child is ready to drink from a glass or tumbler, provide some extra grip by wrapping elastic bands around it.

Feeding utensils

Wash brand new utensils before using them and never use utensils or implements with sharp edges. Choose spoons that have a narrow bowl. Many baby spoons are coated in rubber; if the rubber is torn, throw the spoon away because bacteria can get into the tears. Wash plates and spoons in hot water. Bowls with suction on the bottom can be very difficult to clean. If bowls or plates are made of flexible plastic, clean with salt and wash thoroughly.

Melted spoon in dishwasher

Q: 'I use a lot of plastic spoons feeding my young child and wash them in the dishwasher,' reports Mimi. 'One of the spoons fell onto the heating element and melted. What can I do?'

Problem:	Plastic spoon on dishwasher heating element
What to use:	Professional help
How to apply:	If you can remove the spoon entirely, that's fine, but you have to be very careful with heating elements. If there's even the smallest amount of plastic, it can clog up the moving parts inside the dishwasher. Don't attempt to fix this yourself. Consult a dishwasher repairer.

Pea stains on table

Q: 'When our son was a baby, he used to shove his peas under the table protector (unbeknown to us),' says Tyson. 'So now we have all these green stains over our polished wooden dining table. What can we do?'

Problem:	Pea stains on polished timber
What to use:	Beeswax, or glycerine and talcum powder; cloth; UV light
How to apply:	If the table has a shellac finish, use beeswax on a cloth. If the table has a polyurethane finish, polish with a paste of equal parts glycerine and talcum powder on a cloth. To remove any residual green, expose the stains to sunlight or a UV light.

How to make home-made rusks

Ingredients: 150 g plain flour, 90 g arrowroot (or rice) flour,
½ teaspoon of baking soda, ½ teaspoon of cream of tartar,
5 tablespoons of breast milk or formula, 1 teaspoon of a grain-
based oil, such as canola.

Method: Mix ingredients until stiff. Place baking paper on a
bench. Roll the mixture into large pieces thicker than your
thumb but no more than 2.5 cm thick. Remove air pockets
and rough bits. If the dough is dry, dampen your hands as you
roll. Bake at 180°C until just coloured. This should take 8 to
10 minutes.

How to clean blenders, food grinders and food mills

When your baby starts eating solid foods, your blender will be
in regular use.

To clean

- Heat ½ cup of white vinegar in the microwave until it's
  steaming but not boiling.
- Place the vinegar in the blender and add 2 teaspoons of
  bicarb.
- Switch on the blender for 1 minute. Don't forget to put the
  lid on.
- Rinse thoroughly with water.

Avoid cleaning with detergent because it leaves a residue that's
difficult to remove.

Baby food grinders and food mills that are operated by hand are often easier to clean than electric blenders. They also have the added benefit of portability, so you can purée food away from home. You can make small quantities of food without too much washing up.

DID YOU KNOW? When your baby eats solid food, their poo can look alarming. For example, banana often leaves black specks in poo. If in doubt, get medical advice, but be aware that different foods have different digestive impacts.

CHAPTER 4

BATHING AND
CHANGING

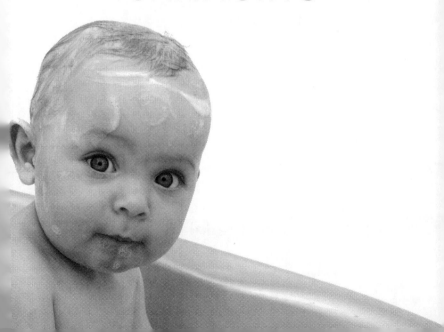

There's nothing as cute as the first time your baby discovers splashing water. And with a little savvy preparation, you can enjoy bath time as well and avoid a mess. When you become used to it, bathing and changing can be fun and a great opportunity to bond. But be warned: there's a lot more splashing when toddlers take a bath.

HOW TO CREATE SOOTHING BATHS

Newborns can be bathed in a small plastic bath or even the kitchen sink. If you use the sink, it must be cleaned thoroughly first. Before bathing baby, place a towel in the bottom of the sink and cover taps or anything the baby could knock their body on with a towel. If using a plastic bath, ensure it's securely placed and won't spill. If there's carpet, put a large non-slip plastic mat in the splash zone (similar to those used in offices, with spikes to hold the mat securely on the carpet – available at hardware stores). Ensure the temperature in the room is warm and only fill the sink or bath with 15 cm of water – enough for the baby to float in but not so much that they can't feel the bottom. Test the water temperature on your wrist in the same way you test the contents of a baby's bottle. It should be blood-heat temperature – 37°C – just shy of cold with a hint of warm. As the water is running over your wrist, look away; if you can't feel hot or cold, it's the ideal temperature. Never use hot water. If your baby's toes turn pink when placed in the water, it's too hot. Never leave your baby unattended while bathing.

It's important for your baby to have good support. If you're not comfortable, the baby won't feel comfortable either. Place your arm underneath the baby's neck and secure your thumb and forefinger around their upper arm furthest from you. That way, their head won't be able to fall from your wrist. This is the most secure grip. Wash them with pH neutral soap (baby soap) or, if the baby's skin is sensitive, sorbolene cream. Wipe the baby with a clean washer. Washing and massaging their head is very important, but there's no need to buy baby shampoo. Just use baby soap and softly massage, into their scalp. This will help to prevent cradle cap.

 TIP If your baby screams when placed in bath water, hold them at the edge of the bath and allow them to play with the water until they become used to it. It's difficult to bathe a baby that has gone stiff.

When it comes to toddlers, be careful of scalding water and slipping. Install childproof taps and adjust the hot water temperature at the thermostat. The optimum temperature for a storage hot water system is 60–65° C in the tank or 50° C in an instantaneous hot water system. A lower temperature at the thermostat will also reduce your power bill. To guard against slipping, place non-slip mats or stickers on the bottom of the bathtub. You can also buy rubber covers for taps to protect little heads. Only fill the bath to the level of your toddler's waist when they are sitting and ensure electrical items and your bath products are out of their reach. Again, never leave children unattended in the bath.

Essential bathing kit for babies

4 cotton baby towels – choose good quality, soft towels that aren't too dense. Dense towels don't mould to a baby or toddler's shape, and they create more fluff, which can irritate their skin. Shannon uses linen towels.

6 cotton flannels – ideal for wiping.

pH neutral soap (baby soap) or sorbolene cream

Baby creams – choose creams that are phthalate free (phthalate is often listed as 'fragrance' on the ingredients list of a product). To prevent chafing, rub cream over the areas where skin contacts skin, such as the crooks of their elbows, the crease in their neck and under their armpits. You only need a small amount (the size of a 10 cent piece). Make sure your hands are clean before applying.

How to clean baby towels

Before using new towels, wash them twice in the washing machine to remove fabric dressing. Ideally, wash them with this homemade laundry detergent for delicate skin.

- Combine 1 tablespoon of pure soap flakes, the juice of 1 lemon and 2 tablespoons of bicarb in a large jar.
- Add 2 cups of warm water, mix well and label the jar.
- For a regular size, lightly soiled load, use 1 tablespoon of this mixture for a top loader and ½ tablespoon for a front loader.
- Hang in the sun to dry – the UV in sunshine is a disinfectant.

Don't use fabric softener in the wash because it can irritate skin and makes nappies less absorbent. Instead, add white vinegar to the fabric conditioner slot.

If your baby has a gassy tummy, give them a gentle massage after their bath. Place a little baby oil or cream on your hand, put your hand flat over their tummy and gently rub in an anticlockwise direction. Massage their feet with the palm of your hand on the outside edge to the arch of the foot. Don't rub too softly, because it tickles – or too strongly, because it's painful. A foot massage can often send a baby to sleep.

You don't need to worry about water spills in the bathroom, but mop up after bathing in other parts of the house. Water on the floor can be slippery and hazardous.

The baby's umbilical stump will fall off about 4 to 7 days after birth. Wipe the area clean with a cloth and only use pH neutral soap. Allow the area to dry before putting on a nappy. Always wash your hands before touching the stump to protect against germs. Once the stump falls off, it will take around 10 days to heal. If you have any concerns, ask at the baby health clinic.

 If your baby has eczema, add 1 teaspoon of medical-grade or Manuka honey (available at pharmacies) to the bath water. This raw, unprocessed honey is an antibacterial, helps with itching and isn't sticky. Proprietary product Pinetarsol also relieves itching. If you use Pinetarsol, wash the bath afterwards because pine oil can affect plastics.

Should you use bubble bath?

Baby skin is very sensitive and bubble bath can be irritating. If you want to use bubble bath, ensure it's created especially for babies and is pH neutral. And if there's any reaction, stop using it.

Should you get a change table with a bath attached?

Bathing a baby in their bedroom isn't always convenient. Think about lugging the water back and forth from the bathroom or kitchen each time. There's a greater likelihood of water spills on the carpet or floor. Also, you tend to stop using the baby bath after 6 months, but use the change table for 2 years.

How to clean a plastic baby bath

After removing the water, wipe over the plastic with equal parts white vinegar and water on a cloth. The acid in white vinegar neutralises soap. Allow the bath to dry outside or under an open window in sunshine to kill bacteria.

CHANGING BABY

Locate the change area away from draughts – you don't want your baby to get a chill. Before bathing, lay out their clothes in the order they'll be put on, making sure you have enough layers in cooler weather. When it's cool, protect your baby's head with a baby cap so they don't get a headache from the cold. Ribbons don't keep their head warm and can be irritating. It also makes them look like an Easter egg.

 TIP If there are lice or bed bugs in the house, add 1 or 2 drops of tea tree oil to the bathwater. Don't rinse the baby's eyes with this water.

DID YOU KNOW? For many years, mothers were encouraged to place babies in morning or afternoon sunlight for 10 minutes, nappy-free, for what's known as 'sun kicks'. *Baby Love* author Robin Barker doesn't think it's necessary in Australia and warns against placing babies in direct sunlight in their first 12 months. During nappy-free time, place a towel underneath your baby; when boys are lying on their backs, a washer can prevent urine spray.

Change mats and tables

A dedicated baby change table is a fantastic investment. The padded top is waterproof, it has a protective edge or securing strap so the baby can't roll off, there are spots for lotions and creams that are in reach for you but out of reach for the baby, and there's plenty of storage underneath for nappies and towels. Shannon used one that was passed around within the family; made from chrome and plastic, it folded into a single column – ideal if you don't have much space. The change table should be safe and comfortable for the baby and high enough that you don't get a backache.

⚠ WARNING

Never take a hand off your baby during changing.
Don't answer the phone or send a text. Turn the cook top
off and don't allow yourself to be interrupted.

 Babies like to wriggle, but if you change their nappy in the same spot each time, they'll associate this area with nappy changing.

Baby foam change mats or change pads

Baby foam change mats or change pads are a 5 cm thick piece of foam with raised, wedged sides, so the baby can safely lie in the dip. They can be placed on many surfaces, including benches. Covered with waterproof vinyl, it's easy to clean these mats or pads with a damp, soapy cloth or white vinegar on a cloth. When using a mat or pad, keep lotions in a small basket within easy reach for you but out of reach for the baby. Covers are available for change mats but are not necessary.

You can always change your baby on the floor – there's nowhere for them to fall. Place a towel or change mat underneath the baby, sit flat on the floor with your legs splayed in a V shape, and place the baby between your legs – they won't be able to roll past your legs.

Without a nappy on, girls' pee goes down but boys' pee goes up, and is able to go long distances. Have white vinegar on hand to remove pee stains when necessary. When changing a boy, lay a clean nappy over his penis as soon as you remove the old nappy so he doesn't pee across the room.

Cloth versus disposable nappies

There's an ongoing debate about the environmental impact of cloth and disposable nappies. A University of Queensland study found disposable nappies use more energy, land area and solid waste, but cloth nappies use more water. There are many biodegradable nappies available for sale in Australia. The most suitable brand will depend on several factors including absorbency, size and price. Try different brands until you find the best one for you.[17] You'll spend up to three times more money on disposable nappies.

Types of cloth nappies

In addition to **cotton** and **terry towelling**, other cloth nappies are available.

Bamboo nappies look like cotton ones but are softer and more absorbent; because they absorb more urine, double the amount of white vinegar you add to the nappy bucket (see page 84 for

---

17 www.choice.com.au/reviews-and-tests/babies-and-kids/kids-health/
nappies/disposable-nappies-review-and-compare/page/nappies%20and%20
the%20environment.aspx

how to clean cloth nappies). For brands that don't recommend cleaning with white vinegar, add a squeeze of fresh lemon juice instead.

Hemp nappies are more absorbent but can become prickly after a few washes, so use a liner.

Merino wool nappies containing lanolin are ideal for newborns. Wool can't be washed in commercial nappy soakers because these contain bleach. Instead, clean with 1 teaspoon of cheap shampoo in a 9 litre bucket of water. Rinse in water and dry in sunshine. You'll also need to replenish the lanolin in the wool every couple of months. To do this, place 1 teaspoon of lanolin in a microwave-safe dish (glass or ceramic, not plastic) with 1 cup of hot water and heat until the lanolin melts. Wring the wool nappies in the solution and dry in sunshine.

 Cloth nappies with liners are better for nappy rash because more air flows through them. Don't use wipes if your baby has nappy rash or reacts to wipes. Shannon prefers to use a damp washer or flannel.

Disposable nappies

It's important to change disposable nappies as soon as they are soiled because urine quickly becomes acidic and can cause nappy rash. Never leave a baby in a wet nappy for more than 10 minutes. Many disposable nappies contain polyacrylate crystals, which turn liquid into gel, to absorb moisture. You need to change the nappy as soon as it's soiled because urine generates fumes that aggravate baby skin.

Barrier creams for nappy rash

If your baby has nappy rash, there are several types of barrier creams. Zinc-based creams prevent urine from penetrating the skin. Papaw ointment acts as a barrier and also soothes the skin. Whatever you use, ensure the cream is removed each day with a damp washer – don't just reapply more cream on top of previous applications. Before using a cream, ask your baby health clinic consultant or chemist for advice on whether it protects and soothes baby skin.

An old-fashioned remedy for nappy rash is to wipe over the affected area with cotton wool balls dipped in a saline solution, followed by a little extra virgin olive oil on the affected area. Be aware that some babies react to olive oil if it contains soybean oil, so test a small area of their skin first. Don't use olive oil if your baby has eczema, and seek professional advice if the rash persists.

Q: 'I accidentally smeared ointment on my cotton shirt,' says Isla. 'Can I remove it?'

Problem:	**Ointment on fabric**
What to use:	**Blood-heat water; cake of bathroom soap, dishwashing liquid; grated soap; tea tree oil; white vinegar**
How to apply:	Remove excess ointment under the tap using blood-heat (body temperature) water. For water-based ointments, scribble with a cake of bathroom soap. Massage with your

fingertips until the stain is loosened. For grey staining, massage with a couple of drops of dishwashing liquid on your fingertips until the liquid feels like jelly. For antibacterial ointments, combine 1 teaspoon of grated bathroom soap, 1 teaspoon of dishwashing liquid and 1 tablespoon of boiling water. Allow the mixture to dissolve. Massage 2 drops of the solution into the stain with your fingertips until the solution feels like jelly. For wax-based ointments, mix 2 drops of tea tree oil with 2 drops of dishwashing liquid and massage with your fingertips until the liquid feels like jelly. For liniment (alcohol-based ointments), blot with or soak in white vinegar. In all cases, wash according to the fabric. Dry on the clothesline or clothes airer.

Nappy rash cream in carpet

Q: 'How can I get lanolin-based nappy rash cream out of our new carpet?' asks Donna.

Problem:	**Nappy rash cream in carpet**
What to use:	**Dishwashing liquid, tea tree oil, cold water, cloth, paper towel; or talcum powder, pantyhose**
How to apply:	Remove excess cream by lifting with a plastic comb or by blotting with paper towel.

For lanolin-based cream, massage with a couple of drops of dishwashing liquid on your fingertips until the liquid feels like jelly. Mix 1 teaspoon of tea tree oil with 1 cup of cold water and wipe on with a cloth. For zinc-based cream, sprinkle with talcum powder and scrub with pantyhose first. Mix 1 teaspoon of tea tree oil with 1 cup of cold water and wipe on with a cloth. Absorb moisture by covering the area with paper towel. Place a book on top of the paper towel to assist with absorption.

 When pinning your baby's nappy, slide your hand between the nappy and the baby's tummy so that if you pin anything, it will be your hand. To dull the ends of nappy pins, rub the sharp point over a cake of bathroom soap. It will then pierce rather than catch the fabric.

What to do with dirty cloth nappies

Place dirty cloth nappies in a lidded, sealed bucket. To clean, use two buckets.

■ Fill one bucket ¾ full of water and add Shannon's nappy soaker. Make this by mixing 1 teaspoon of 3 per cent hydrogen peroxide and 1 teaspoon of homemade laundry detergent (1 tablespoon of pure soap flakes, the juice of 1 lemon, 2 tablespoons of bicarb and 2 cups of warm water, mixed well in a large jar.)

- Fill a second bucket with hot water and 1 teaspoon of tea tree oil.
- Shake any solids from the nappy into the toilet.
- Rinse the nappy under water.
- Place nappies in the first bucket and leave for 12 hours.
- Place nappies in the second bucket and leave for 20 minutes.
- Wash in the washing machine with hot water and 1 teaspoon of *Vanish NapiSan Oxi Action Sensitive Powder* or ¼ cup bicarb.
- Add ½ cup of white vinegar to the fabric conditioner slot.
- Dry in the sun.

If you like to wash with bicarb, white vinegar or essential oils but are using modern cloth nappies, check that these ingredients won't affect the nappies' elasticity. Don't be seduced by products with antibacterial properties: these aren't necessary when cleaning nappies. It's best to dry nappies on a clothesline in the sun, which both sterilises and fades stains. It's also gentler on the nappy fibres, so nappies will last longer. If you have to use the clothes dryer, iron the nappies afterwards to kill any bacteria.

 Absorb nasty odours and release a pleasant fragrance by mixing 2 tablespoons of bicarb, ½ teaspoon of dried sage, ½ teaspoon of dried thyme and 2 drops of lavender oil in a saucer. Place this mixture near the nappy bucket. Never overfill a nappy bucket, because waste could run down its side and onto the carpet.

More is not better

Don't overuse lotions and creams. More is not better and in
some cases, overuse can be dangerous. Lotions are a mixture
of water and oil, along with emulsifiers that stop the product
from separating. Choose products based on the ingredients list,
rather than on words such as 'pure' or 'gentle' on the packaging.
Ingredients are listed in descending order of mass or volume
– the first item in the list has the highest mass or volume. In
Australia, the National Industrial Chemicals Notification and
Assessment Scheme (NICNAS) has a cosmetic standard that
can be viewed online. And remember, the natural oils in your
baby's skin are usually all they need.[18]

How to change a nappy

- Assemble everything you need in the order you need it:
  - changing mat
  - nappy, nappy liner, safety pins and pilchers (if using a
    cloth nappy)
  - cotton wool
  - baby oil
  - cream
  - damp washer
- Remove the dirty nappy and use the front part to wipe off as
  much poo as you can. Fold the dirty nappy in two and slide
  the clean side underneath the baby's bottom.

---

18 http://www.nicnas.gov.au/chemical-information/cosmetics

- Clean the baby with a damp washer.
- Put on a clean nappy. Dress the baby.
- Put the dirty cloth nappy in the bucket or the disposable nappy in the bin. Wash your hands.

Different poos and how to clean them

You'll see a whole range of poo with different colours, consistencies and smells. Some will look like mustard seeds, others like peanut butter. Your baby's first poo is called meconium; it's olive in colour, tar-like in consistency and very high in protein. Poo produced after drinking breast milk and formula is also high in protein. To clean, rinse under cold water. Never use hot water on a protein stain because it will set. Wash in the washing machine on a cold setting. The best way to remove poo stains from fabric is with sunshine – the UV rays in sunshine fade stains. Avoid using the dryer unless you have to. If you can, wash first thing in the morning to maximise exposure to sunshine.

Cleaning urine stains

The other common stain is urine, which is removed with white vinegar. Blot or soak the stain with white vinegar and wash normally.

Disposable nappy in washing machine or dryer

Q: 'I never would have done this if I'd had enough sleep,' says Melissa. 'But I accidentally put a disposable nappy in the washing machine. How can I fix the melted mess?'

Problem:	**Disposable nappy through washing machine or dryer**
What to use:	**Hair conditioner, bicarb, water, pantyhose (washing machine); glycerine, pantyhose (dryer)**
How to apply:	Allow the washing machine drum to fill with water, then add 2 tablespoons of cheap hair conditioner and 2 tablespoons of bicarb. Leave the machine filled for 1 hour before rinsing and wiping out with pantyhose. To fix the dryer, empty and wipe the cold drum with glycerine on pantyhose. Shake all the affected clothes thoroughly before rewashing.

Pilchers

Pilchers are placed over cloth nappies to protect against leakage. They are available in different fabrics and plastics. Avoid plastic or PUL (polyurethane laminate) pilchers before 6 months. Instead, use woollen pilchers that expand with moisture but still allow airflow. Pilchers also come in polyester fleece that wicks away moisture. Change them when you change the nappy.

To clean plastic and PUL pilchers

- Wash thoroughly with a cake of bathroom soap and cold water.

- Hang in sunshine to dry.

Don't soak PUL pilchers in nappy soakers; it makes them brittle.

To clean wool pilchers

- Wash thoroughly in cold water with a cake of bathroom soap. Don't use hot water, because it will shrink the wool fibres.
- Hang in sunshine. Turn them inside out so the sunlight sanitises both sides.

To clean fleece pilchers

- Wash in the washing machine using ½ teaspoon of laundry detergent, bicarb and white vinegar.
- If the pilchers are lined with rubber, turn them inside out as they dry so sunshine hits both sides of the pilchers.

How to fold cloth nappies

In the first months, fold the nappy to create a triangle, then fold again. Place the longest side in line with the baby's waist and pull the pointed part through their legs. Secure with safety pins. The most common nappy fold is the kite – lay the nappy flat and fold the two sides so they meet in the middle. Then pull the top flap over the top to create an envelope. Another option is to fold two peaks top and bottom first, then fold the sides. This means less folded material against the baby and ensures better poo catching. It can expand as the baby grows. See page 237 for a diagram.

 Make life easier for yourself by pre-folding nappies. Store them in a nappy hanger.

How to make a baby nappy hanger

What you need: old pillowcase, piece of cardboard 12 cm x
9 cm, needle, thread, coat-hanger

Method: Lay the pillowcase flat with the opening away
from you. Cut one layer of the fabric down the centre. Sew
bias binding along the cut edges to make it smooth. Wrap
cardboard in plastic or fabric and place in the bottom of the cut
pillowcase. Fold the corners over it and stitch into position. In
the top flap, make a hole and place a coat-hanger inside. The
hanger protects from dust and is easy to access. You can make
several.

Nappy wipes

Although nappy wipes are convenient and easy to carry,
many babies are allergic to the chemicals used in them.
Shannon prefers to use a damp washer with a little baby
soap. Keep wipes handy for emergencies only and to remove
the bulk of muck.

 For awful nappy-changing smells, mix 2 drops of lavender
oil in 1 litre of water in a spray pack and spray the air in
the room. Keep a small vial of lavender oil in your nappy
bag. Buy the cheapest lavender oil because it's lower
in fragrance and higher in volatiles, which act as an
antibacterial agent.

Recycle old cloth nappies – the cotton is great quality. Shannon often buys old ones at garage sales to use as cleaning rags. Turn them into washers – they are soft enough to wash a baby's face or bottom. If they have only been peed on, reuse disposable nappies in the garden to protect seedlings. When planting, place a used disposable nappy in the bottom of a dug-out hole, and place the plant on top. The nappy will work like water crystals and help retain water.

Stubborn nappy stains

Q: 'How do I get poo stains from a breast-fed baby out of light-coloured clothes?' asks Michelle.

Problem:	**Poo stains in fabric**
What to use:	**Cold water, cake of bathroom soap, dishwashing liquid, sunshine; or glycerine or bicarb, cold water, sunshine**
How to apply:	Remove excess poo under the tap using cold water. Scribble stain with a cake of bathroom soap run under cold water. Massage with a couple of drops of dishwashing liquid on your fingertips until the liquid feels like jelly. Rinse using cold water. If there are colourants, wipe with 2 drops of glycerine and leave for 90 minutes. Alternatively, soak overnight in cold water and ¼ cup of bicarb. In both cases,

wash according to the fabric. Dry in sunshine to fade remaining stains.

Problem: **Diarrhoea in clothing**

What to use: **Cold water, cake of bathroom soap, dishwashing liquid; or *Vanish NapiSan Oxi Action Sensitive Powder*, bucket; or bicarb**

How to apply: Remove excess poo under the tap using cold water. Scribble with a cake of bathroom soap run under cold water. Massage with a couple of drops of dishwashing liquid on your fingertips until the liquid feels like jelly. Rinse using cold water. Alternatively, mix ½ lid of *Vanish NapiSan Oxi Action Sensitive Powder* in a 9 litre bucket of cold water and soak for 20 minutes. Or soak overnight in a bucket of cold water with ¼ cup of bicarb. In all cases, wash according to the fabric. Dry in sunshine.

 TIP If you notice a reaction in your breastfed baby after you eat mouldy cheeses, inform your baby health clinic or doctor. It could be a sign they are allergic to penicillin.

Potty training

Children's digestion is faster than adults', so place them on the potty after eating but don't let them sit on it for more than 5 minutes at a time. If you do, they'll see the potty as punishment. Instead, read a short story to them to help them relax. To clean the potty, pour the contents into the toilet and flush, wipe the potty with white vinegar on a cloth and, when possible, leave it in sunshine to dry. Rinse with water.

 If you have toilet training steps, ensure they are secure. Wipe regularly with lavender spray on a cloth.

 If your boy is having difficulty getting all his pee in the toilet bowl, put a ping-pong ball inside the bowl and have him aim at it. You can even draw a smiley face on it – he can try to sink the :-). The ping-pong ball won't flush because it's too light, and you'll be surprised at how much better his aim becomes.

 To remove Band-Aids, wipe over the Band-Aid with baby oil or tea tree oil on a cotton ball. Tea tree oil is more effective, but some babies' and toddlers' skin can react to it.

OLD-FASHIONED REMEDIES FOR COMMON FIRST-AID PROBLEMS

An old-fashioned remedy for **intestinal threadworms** is to eat grated carrot and drink carrot juice. This works particularly well with children. If you think your child has threadworm, give them a warm bath before bed and, once they are asleep, take a torch and look at their backside. The worms come out at night. Prevent worms by teaching children to wash their hands, especially after playing with animals. For tapeworms and flatworms, consult a doctor.

To remove a shallow splinter, rub sideways with a blunt probe. If it's deep, but there is sufficient splinter sticking out of the skin, use tweezers in line with the splinter. For a surface splinter, use the eye of a needle, not the point. Put the splinter through the eye of the needle, twist and pull. For persistent splinters, place ¼ teaspoon of *Vegemite* over the splinter and cover with a *Band-Aid* or bandage. The yeast in *Vegemite* forms a poultice that draws the splinter to the surface of the skin.

For a child's (but not a young baby's) cough or cold, wrap a tissue around some sage and thyme and secure it with an elastic band. Put this inside their pillowcase and they'll sleep better.

For a child's (but not a baby's) bronchial cough or wheeze, take 2 whole nutmegs and pierce them end to end with a bodkin. Thread a piece of ribbon through both nutmegs and hang around your child's neck. Encourage them to spin the beads along the string. Nutmeg is a bronchial dilator and raises adrenalin levels.

To lessen the **smell of vomit**, put a ring of toothpaste on the inside rim of the vomit bucket. Peppermint also settles the stomach.

If using **calamine lotion** on children, draw it on with a cotton bud to create flowers or aeroplanes – they'll think it's fun.

Everyone hates **nits**. It's such a problem in Australia that researchers estimate that 10–40 per cent of school children currently have lice. Proprietary products are available but are often very harsh (especially on sensitive scalps) and Shannon has found that head lice become immune to most of them, one by one. This means you can end up using one product after another, trying to find the one that your local lice are not immune to. Shannon recommends applying unsweetened orange juice to the hair and using a nit comb to comb out the eggs. Add a couple of drops of tea tree oil to shampoos and conditioners and to bathwater to prevent them. No matter which solution you use, you must comb out every nit. A researcher at James Cook University suggests applying conditioner to dry hair, covering each strand of hair from root to tip. Detangle the hair with an ordinary comb. Then immediately comb the hair with a fine-toothed comb or plastic nit comb. Wipe the conditioner from the fine-toothed comb onto a tissue and look for lice and eggs. Repeat the combing for every part of the head at least five times. Head lice die once they leave the head.

For regular **childhood nosebleeds**, place a chilled cloth on the back of the child's neck and pinch the bridge of the nose with your fingers. If the bleeding doesn't stop in 5 minutes or is very fast, seek medical aid. Never put a child's head back while their nose is bleeding because they can drown in their own blood. Encourage them to breathe through their mouth.

To cure **hiccups**, drink a teaspoon of white vinegar and force yourself to shudder. This causes the vinegar to bubble in your throat and confuses the nervous system. Once you confuse the nervous system, you'll stop hiccupping.

To soothe the **itching from sandflies**, mix equal parts cold tea and methylated spirits or dab a little white vinegar on the bites. A paste of bicarb and water also works, but don't use this on children under the age of 2 years because their skin could react to the bicarb.

To **relieve sunburn**, have a cool but not hot shower and apply the prescription cream Silvadene. Aloe vera gel is also soothing for burns, although some people are allergic to it. Rub a cut tomato over the burn for temporary relief.

To **get rid of warts**, apply white sap from a dandelion plant but only to the wart itself or you will burn the surrounding skin. There are many old wives' tales about removing warts and they're all fanciful. One such remedy was to rub a piece of meat over the wart and bury the meat in the garden. As the meat rotted, the wart was supposed to magically fall off. It doesn't work.

Relieve the **itching of chickenpox** by applying mint tea to the skin. Or add several mint tea bags to a cool bath.

CHAPTER 5

CLOTHING AND LAUNDRY

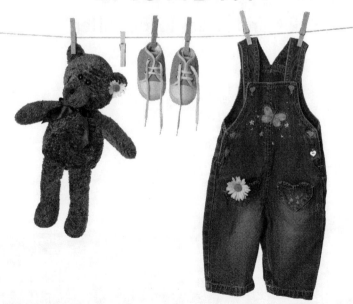

Baby and toddler clothing is super cute. Those tiny singlets, jumpsuits, dresses and overalls – not to mention booties – are adorable. But remember: you'll be changing and washing them over and over, so choose items that are easy to care for. Also think about your baby's comfort and opt for natural fibres – they are better for their skin and easier to look after.

HOW TO CHOOSE BABY CLOTHING

Babies can't tell you if their clothing is uncomfortable, so feel inside new garments with the back of your hand. Even if the clothing is made from 100 per cent cotton, it could be stitched using polyester thread, which can be irritating. Shannon's mum used to run her tongue along the inside of the necks and arms of clothing checking for scratchiness. If there's roughness, sew cotton bias binding or iron-on cotton hemming tape over the seam. Fold the edges of the hemming tape underneath so there are no stiff gluey bits.

Here are Shannon's suggestions when shopping for baby clothes.

- Avoid baby clothing that has buttons down the back. They are uncomfortable for the baby to lie on.
- Choose clothing that is easy to put on and take off.
- Avoid white items – they show stains more easily.
- Clothing should never leave a mark on your baby's skin. If this happens, it's time for a bigger size.
- It's best not to use clothing made of polyester fabric. If you do, clean it with cheap hair shampoo because soap flakes can remove the chemical flame-retardant that's added to some baby sleepwear.

Sizing

Babies grow at different rates, so choose clothes according to the child's weight, not their age. As a general rule, a 3 kilogram baby will be size 00000, a 4 kilogram baby size 0000, a

6 kilogram baby (3-6 months) size 000, an 8 kilogram baby (3-6 months) size 00, a 10 kilogram baby (6-12 months) size 0, a 12 kilogram baby (12-18 months) size 1, and a 14 kilogram baby (18-24 months) size 2.

Essential clothing for babies

These items should see you through the first few months.

- 10 singlets or singlet suits – 100 per cent cotton. Be careful with woollens, which may feel soft to an adult but can be prickly on baby skin.
- 4 each of long sleeved and short sleeved bodysuits – as close to 100 per cent cotton as possible
- 4 pairs of short and long cotton pants
- 4 long sleeved tops/jumpers – choose ones with shoulder fastenings or buttons down the front. Babies don't like to have tight clothing pulled over their heads, but they need a snug fit for warmth
- 2 matching outfits for going out – if they match, you can swap a dirty piece with a clean one and no one will be the wiser
- 2 jackets – not too heavy or stiff
- 4 all-in-one outfits – cotton, not terry towelling or flannelette
- 2 cotton hats
- 1 or 2 pairs of cotton mittens – great to keep little fingers warm and to prevent the baby from scratching their face while sleeping
- Numerous pairs of socks – they always get lost. Choose cotton socks that reach above the ankle. If they are all the same colour, you won't have to worry about missing socks.

■ 2 or 3 sleeping outfits. You can use all-in-ones/wonder suits or 'sleeping bags' – nightgowns that are stitched or have drawstring across the bottom so little feet don't get cold.

Dress your baby for comfort and according to the weather. During summer, you'll need more sleeveless items. Shannon also suggests using bunny rugs made from gauze, which are light and cool. In cooler weather, warm your baby with brushed cotton or cotton waffle. Dress with layers of clothing rather than heavy clothes so you can add or remove layers as needed. As a guide, dress your baby or toddler in one more layer than you're wearing – they feel fluctuations in the weather more than adults do.

TIP When putting tops and T-shirts over your baby's head, scrunch the fabric up to the hole and place it at the back of your baby's head, then quickly pull the front over their face. To remove, reverse the process. When removing, take their arms out first and then pull the shirt over your baby's head.

TIP Many baby garments are secured with drawstrings or ribbons. It's important they are stitched securely, not just threaded, because if the drawstrings or ribbons are pulled out, they are a potential choking hazard.

HOW TO WASH BABY CLOTHING

Until your baby is 6 months old, it's preferable to wash their clothes separately from the household wash. Always wash new clothing before your baby wears it to remove fabric dressing and chemicals because baby skin is very sensitive. For any hand-me-down clothing that is stained, soak in cold water and scrub with a cake of bathroom soap before washing. Consult the A–Z guide at the back of this book for spot cleaning. The important part of washing is rinsing in order to remove as much soap as possible.

It'll all come out in the wash

Check that your washing machine is working efficiently:

- Clean the dispenser slots in soapy water.
- Wipe over seals with a cloth. To prevent mould, wipe with a cloth sprayed with ¼ teaspoon of oil of cloves in a 1-litre spray pack of water.
- Once a month, run an empty load using hot water and 2 cups of white vinegar.
- Ensure the washer is level and adjust the legs if necessary. If the floor surface is slippery, use non-slip pads under the feet of the washing machine.
- Each week, wipe over the drum with a cloth wrung in white vinegar.
- Clear the lint catcher regularly. In top loaders, it's located on top of the agitator, or in a bag on the side of the drum. New machines generally have automatic lint cleaners. Consult the instructions.
- If there's a smell, check the pipes. They are easy to replace.
- Have your washing machine serviced every 12 months (every 6 months with a baby).

TIP To test the efficiency of your washing machine, place a small amount of vegetable dye or food colouring on a cotton cloth and allow it to dry. Then wash it (on its own) in the washing machine. If all the colouring comes out in the wash, your washing machine is working well.

Can I use regular detergent?

When your baby is under 6 months, use only the mildest detergents. Baby laundry detergents are available but can be quite expensive. A cheaper, but still effective option is to use 1 tablespoon of pure soap flakes in the washing slot and 2 tablespoons of white vinegar in the fabric conditioner slot of the washing machine. Or try Shannon's DIY delicates laundry detergent recipe.

Shannon's DIY delicates laundry detergent

- Combine 1 tablespoon of pure soap flakes, 2 tablespoons of lemon juice and 2 tablespoons of bicarb in a large jar. Add 2 cups of warm water and mix well.
- Label the jar.
- For a regular size lightly soiled load, use 1 tablespoon of this mixture for a top loader and ½ tablespoon for a front loader.
- Hang clothing in the sun to dry

In terms of stain-removing soakers, there's a commercial formulation for sensitive skin called *Vanish NapiSan Oxi Action Sensitive Powder* that doesn't contain enzymes, dyes or fragrances. Check your baby's skin for any rashes or reactions and don't continue to use it if their skin is affected.

After 6 months, it's fine to use regular laundry detergent, but Shannon suggests using half the amount recommended by the manufacturer. If you're concerned that regular laundry detergent may be too harsh on your baby's skin, wash and dry a couple of baby items with the detergent, dress your baby in them and check their skin for signs of irritation. If there's a rash, don't use the detergent. Instead, use 2 teaspoons of cheap shampoo mixed with 2 tablespoons of bicarb in place of laundry detergent and add 2 tablespoons of white vinegar to the fabric conditioner slot (never use fabric conditioner).

 Liquid laundry detergent is less abrasive than powder and creates less soap build-up. If you use powder, dissolve it in water before adding it to the washing slot. Wear rubber gloves when working with enzyme products, which can be harsh on your skin.

What about bleach?

This is one of Shannon's bugbears. She is not a fan of bleach because it's full of chemicals including dioxins, which produce environmental pollutants. It's also harsher on clothing fibres, making them wear more quickly. Bleach on hard surfaces, such as baths, breaks down the surface, making it more porous and susceptible to bacteria. If using bleach, be very careful and don't inhale the fumes. And remember: the sun is a natural bleaching agent.

Preventing baby clothes from shrinking

Q: 'How do I prevent clothing from shrinking?' asks Liv. 'I'm worried the newborn clothes will shrink.'

A: Shrinkage happens when the temperature of the wash water is different from the temperature of the rinse water. If you can, set the thermostat on your washing machine to 37°C – blood-heat temperature. Be careful washing woollens – hand wash in blood-heat water and rinse in blood-heat water. Clothes can become stiff if you use too much laundry detergent or if they are not rinsed well. Add white vinegar to the fabric conditioner slot (never use fabric conditioner).

 If drying baby clothes in a dryer, iron these items as well. Iron steam is hotter than dryer air and kills more bacteria, which means less likelihood of nappy rash. Clean the filter every time you use the dryer. And don't use fabric softener or fragrance cloths in the dryer; the chemicals they contain can irritate baby's skin.

 A squeeze of lemon juice in the rinse water whitens clothes.

How to clean hand-me-down clothes

Hand-me-down clothes are fantastic and often in great condition. No matter who gave them to you and how fastidious they are with cleanliness, it's a good idea to wash all second-hand clothes before your baby or toddler wears them. Wash according to the fabric and dry in sunshine. To remove stains, consult the A–Z Stain Removal guide at the back of this book.

 Don't leave clothes to soak for more than 12 hours. Only soak delicates for 30 minutes. Never soak woollens for more than 20 minutes because the fibres shrink as the water cools.

How to clean in a front-loading washing machine

■ Use ⅛ of the recommended quantity of laundry detergent and 2 tablespoons of bicarb in the washing slot, and 2 tablespoons of white vinegar in the fabric conditioner slot. The best temperature is 37°C – blood-heat water.

How to clean in a top-loading washing machine

■ Combine ¼ of the recommended quantity of laundry detergent with 2 tablespoons of bicarb in the washing slot and 2 tablespoons of white vinegar in the fabric conditioner slot. Best temperature is 37°C – blood-heat (body temperature) water.

TIP To kill bacteria, add ¼ teaspoon of tea tree oil to the fabric conditioner slot of the washing machine. Tea tree oil is a great anti-fungal and especially helpful with nappy rash. Never apply tea tree oil directly to the skin.

A QUICK GUIDE TO REMOVING FOOD STAINS FROM FABRIC

Apple – Wipe with glycerine, leave for 90 minutes. Wash normally.

Avocado – After removing excess, massage with a couple of drops of dishwashing liquid on your fingers until the liquid feels like jelly. Wash normally.

Banana – Wipe with glycerine, leave for 90 minutes. Wash normally.

Blueberries – Blot or soak in white vinegar. Wash normally. Hang in sunshine (UV light fades stains).

Breast milk – Rinse with cold water, scribble with a cake of bathroom soap and rub the fabric against itself using your hands. Wash normally.

Carbohydrates – Carbohydrate stains are darker in the centre, lighter around the edge and feel stiff. To remove sugar stains, including soft drinks, use blood-heat (body temperature) water and scribble with a cake of bathroom soap. Rub the fabric against itself to loosen the stain. Wash according to the fabric. To remove starchy stains, use cold water and follow the same steps. If in doubt, use cold water first.

Carrot – Blot or soak in white vinegar. Wash normally. Hang in sunshine (UV light fades stains).

Cereal – Scribble with a cake of bathroom soap and rinse in blood-heat (body temperature) water. Wash normally.

Custard – Scribble with a cake of bathroom soap and cold water, then rub the fabric against itself using your hands. If there is any residue, massage the fabric with a couple of drops of dishwashing liquid on your fingertips until the liquid feels like jelly. Wash normally and hang in sunshine.

Egg – Scribble with a cake of bathroom soap and rinse in blood-heat (body temperature) water. Wash normally.

Fats/oils – These spread evenly across a surface, feel greasy between your fingers and, if you wash the stained garment, continue to spread. To remove cooking oils, massage the fabric with dishwashing liquid on your fingertips until the liquid feels like jelly. This means the oil has been emulsified and is water soluble. Wipe with a damp cloth.

Milk – Rinse with cold water and a cake of bathroom soap and wash normally.

Pear – Wipe with glycerine, then leave for 90 minutes. Wash normally.

Peas – Blot or soak with white vinegar. Wash normally.

Proteins – These stains have a dark ring around the edge and include blood, seeds, nuts, meat, cheese, milk, other dairy and fish. To remove, use cold water and scribble with a cake of bathroom soap. Rub the fabric against itself to loosen the stain. Wash according to the fabric. Don't use blood-heat (body temperature) or hot water, or you'll set the stain.

Pumpkin – Blot or soak in white vinegar. Wash normally. Hang in sunshine (UV light fades stains).

Sunscreen – Massage with 2 drops of dishwashing liquid with your fingers, then wash with warm water.

Sweet potato – Scribble with a cake of bathroom soap. Wash normally.

Tomato purée – Blot or soak in white vinegar. Wash normally. Hang in sunshine (UV light fades stains).

Watermelon – Becomes alcoholic very quickly, causing a smell. Sponge with white vinegar and sprinkle with bicarb to remove the stain and the smell.

Problem:	**Baby snot on clothing**
What to use:	**Cake of bathroom soap, warm water**
How to apply:	Baby snot can be difficult to remove from clothes. Scribble with a cake of bathroom soap and warm water and rub the fabric against itself. Wash according to the fabric. Make sure you wash your hands thoroughly afterwards.

How to save time sorting and folding

Save time sorting and folding washing by hanging it on the line in sections. When Shannon's children were young, she had one quarter of the clothesline for nappies, one quarter for pants, one quarter for shirts and one quarter for bunny rugs, towels, sheets and flannels. Have two washing baskets and fold clothes as you remove them from the clothesline. It makes the process much quicker and easier.

If there's limited sunshine on the day you do the washing, halfway through drying, turn the clothes on the line upside down. They'll dry more quickly.

HOW TO STORE CLOTHING

■ **Use acid-free drawer liners to prevent yellowing on clothes.** There is a perception that drawer liners are very last century, but Shannon thinks they're great protection for clothes. You can either buy liners or make your own. To make your own drawer liners, buy acid-free paper from an art supplies shop. Fill a spray bottle with warm water, add 1 tea bag, and leave for 3 minutes. Remove the tea bag and add 2 drops of oil of cloves and 2 drops of your favourite essential oil or perfume, then spray over the paper. Allow the paper to dry, cut it to size and place inside drawers. Replace once a year. Clean the inside of drawers with white vinegar on a cloth.

■ **Hang chalk sticks inside wardrobes to absorb moisture.** Tie 6 sticks of white blackboard chalk with string or ribbon and leave inside the wardrobe to absorb moisture. When the chalk sticks are damp, place them in the sunshine to dry out. If you have built-in wardrobes, double the quantity of chalk. If you have stand-alone wardrobes, place them 2 cm from the wall so air flows behind. You can use the chalk over and over again. Wipe interior wardrobe walls with ¼ teaspoon of oil of cloves in a 250 ml bottle of baby oil on a cloth. Re-label the bottle.

For serious continuous damp, seek professional advice
to find the source of the problem, rather than repeatedly
treating only the symptom.

■ **Wipe down mouldy walls.** Mix ¼ teaspoon of oil of cloves
in a 1 litre spray pack of water. Spray onto a cloth and wipe
over walls.

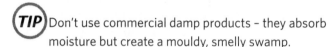 **TIP** Don't use commercial damp products – they absorb
moisture but create a mouldy, smelly swamp.

■ **Store items in regular use at waist height.**
■ **If there's not much space, use open shelves.** Place a
bed sheet over the top of open shelves to prevent dust, or
use a cotton shoe hanger or nappy bag holder to store baby
clothes. Canvas shelving units are a great option because
they allow good airflow and are washable.

How to protect baby clothes for longer-term storage

Before storing, make sure the clothing is completely clean
or mould and mildew will grow. Use acid-free tissue paper
between each layer of clothing to prevent yellow spots. When
an item sweats in plastic, the smallest amount of bacteria
can grow, so it's best not to store baby clothes in plastic bags;
no matter how well items are laundered, they will go yellow
and become smelly. Instead, store clothes in an old cotton
pillowcase that has been boiled in hot water. Store with a cake
of soap or wardrobe sachet. Soap counteracts the tannic acid

in timber and prevents browning in fabric. If using vacuum storage bags, prevent yellowing by placing clothes into clean boiled pillowcases first.

Stained baby shawl

Q: 'My son's baby shawl has been packed away for 30 years,' reports Sue. 'I recently unwrapped it to find a dark yellow stain on it. What can I do?'

Problem:	**Dark yellow stain on baby shawl**
What to use:	**Methylated spirits; or *Vanish NapiSan Oxi Action Sensitive Powder* and blood-heat water; or cheap shampoo, 3 per cent hydrogen peroxide, blood-heat water, bucket**
How to apply:	The stain is likely to be old milk. For synthetic fibres, dip in methylated spirits and wring out tightly. For natural fibres (but not wool or silk), soak overnight in ½ lid of *Vanish NapiSan Oxi Action Sensitive Powder* and 9 litres of blood-heat (body temperature) to hot water. In both cases, wash according to the fabric. Dry in sunshine. For wool, soak in 1 teaspoon of cheap shampoo and 1 tablespoon of 3 per cent hydrogen peroxide in 9 litres of blood-heat (body temperature) water for 20 minutes. Place a dinner plate

on top to keep the item immersed. Rinse in blood-heat water. Gently wring and dry flat on a towel in the shade.

Baby and toddler footwear

Choose shoes that can be washed easily, including cotton and canvas, with good grip on the bottom. Ensure the drawstrings on woollen booties are stitched into position so they can't be pulled out. Babies have a habit of sucking on drawstrings and they could be a choking hazard. For shoes that can't be washed in the washing machine, wipe inside and outside with lavender spray. Feel inside the shoe for any roughness and remove by filing with a nail file.

Toddlers aren't very good at telling you when shoes don't fit well. To work out if shoes are too tight, put dark socks on the child's foot and dust the inside of their shoes with talcum powder. When you remove the shoes, you will see where the pressure points are. When buying shoes, take an old pair of white socks and place some carbon paper inside the sock, carbon-side down. Then try the shoes on. The carbon paper will leave marks on the socks to show how tight the fit is. If the marks are even, the shoes fit well. If there's heavy marking in particular areas, the fit is tight and blisters will form. Wash the socks in milk to remove the carbon ink.

Pee in toddler's shoes

Q: 'My toddler has just moved on from nappies. He's going pretty well, but sometimes he gets really excited, forgets there's no nappy and pees. The problem is that the urine runs into his shoes and smells awful. Is there anything I can do?' asks Matthew.

Problem:	**Urine on shoes**
What to use:	**White spirits, cotton ball, talcum powder, lemon juice, cloth**
How to apply:	Dab the stain with white spirits on a cotton ball and sprinkle with talcum powder inside and outside the shoe. Allow to dry and then brush out. To neutralise the smell, wipe with lemon juice on a cloth. Cloth and vinyl shoes can be washed in the washing machine or hand washed and dried in sunshine.

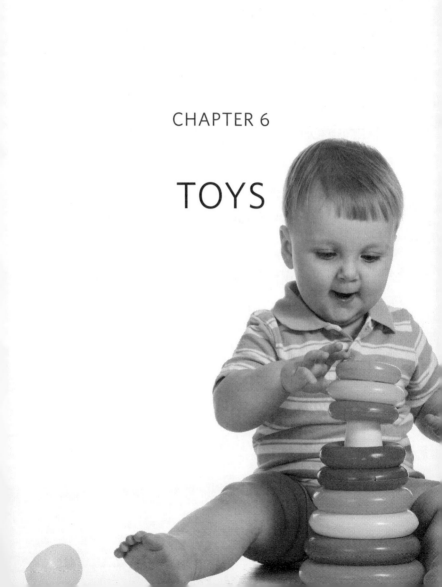

CHAPTER 6

TOYS

Babies and toddlers don't need to have many toys. According to Oliver James, psychologist and author of *Love Bombing*, most children only need a transition object – like their first teddy bear that they take everywhere. Everything else is a socially generated want.[19] Choose toys that encourage play, creativity and imagination and don't feel guilty if your child doesn't have the latest gimmicky one.

19 www.bbc.com/news/magazine-24759728

HOW TO CLEAN TOYS

As a rule, clean all toys before they are used, including soft ones, because you can't be sure where they've been. Even if brand new, many items sit on container terminals where rats and other nasty creepy crawlies wander. For a quick clean, mix ¼ teaspoon of tea tree oil in 1 litre of water in a spray pack, spray onto a cloth and wipe over toys. Carry this mixture with you to use on toys when away from home – in doctor's waiting rooms, for example. Tea tree oil is a disinfectant and is non-toxic.

Problem:	**Dirty hard toy**
What to use:	**Tea tree oil, water, spray pack, cloth; oil of cloves, bucket, blood-heat water**
How to apply:	Mix ¼ teaspoon of tea tree oil in 1 litre of water in a spray pack. Spray over the toy and wipe with a cloth.

Problem:	**Mouldy rubber toy**
What to use:	**Oil of cloves, blood-heat (body temperature) water**
How to apply:	Add ¼ teaspoon of oil of cloves to a 4 litre bucket of blood-heat (body temperature) water. Place the toy in the bucket, squeeze so water gets inside and leave for 2 hours. Remove, squeeze out the water and set aside to dry.

Problem: **Dirty plastic toy**

What to use: **Glycerine, cloth, cake of bathroom soap, cold water, tea tree oil, spray pack**

How to apply: For a new toy, after unwrapping the toy, wipe over the plastic with glycerine on a cloth, then wash with a cake of bathroom soap and cold water. Don't use dishwashing liquid because it can break down petrochemicals. Alternatively, mix ¼ teaspoon of tea tree oil in a 1 litre spray pack of water and wipe over the plastic.

Problem: **Plastic or wooden toys coated in wax**

What to use: **Tea tree oil, glycerine, water, spray pack, pantyhose**

How to apply: Many toys are coated in wax to make them appear shiny. To remove the wax, mix 1 teaspoon of tea tree oil, 1 teaspoon of glycerine and 1 litre of water in a spray pack. Spray onto a pair of pantyhose and wipe over the toy.

TIP In February 2011, the Australian Competition and Consumer Commission introduced a permanent ban on children's plastic products with more than 1 per cent DEHP (diethylhexyl phthalate).

Problem: **Dirty soft toys**
What to use: **Plastic bag, freezer, washing machine, cheap shampoo, tea tree oil, pillowcase, sunshine; or unprocessed wheat bran, white vinegar, scrubbing brush**
How to apply: Place the toy in a plastic bag and put it in the freezer for 12 hours. This kills microscopic bugs and dust mites (although not allergens). Most toys can be washed in the washing machine on a gentle cycle – check the label first. Rather than laundry detergent, use 1 tablespoon of cheap shampoo and 2 drops of tea tree oil to kill dust mites. Place in a delicates bag or pillowcase. Don't use the clothes dryer but hang the toys to dry in sunshine. Alternatively, after removing the soft toy from the freezer, mix 1 kilo of unprocessed wheat bran with several drops of white vinegar until the mixture resembles breadcrumbs. Place inside a pillowcase and add the soft toy. Tie off and shake well. Remove the toy from the pillowcase and brush with a scrubbing brush. If your child has allergies, clean soft toys every month and dry in the sun.

TIP Check that the seams on stuffed toys are strong or stuffing could come out. Ensure there are no sharp, pointy bits on toys.

Problem: **Dirty wooden toys**
What to use: **Tea tree oil, water, spray pack**
How to apply: Spray with ¼ teaspoon of tea tree oil in 1 litre of water in a spray pack. Timber contains an antibacterial agent.

(TIP) Wooden toys, such as blocks, are safest if unvarnished. Varnish flakes are like little pieces of plastic and can become a choking issue if chewed.

Problem: **Dirty metal toys**
What to use: **Baby oil, pantyhose**
How to apply: Place 2 drops of baby oil onto a pair of pantyhose and wipe over the toy. This cleans the toy and stops it from rusting.

Problem: **Grass stains on soft toys**
What to use: **White spirits, cloth; or egg white, glycerine, water**
How to apply: Wipe with white spirits on a cloth. Alternatively, mix equal parts egg white and glycerine to form a soapy paste. The egg white and glycerine need to be at the same temperature, so remove the eggs from the fridge and bring to room temperature. Apply the paste to the stain and leave for one day. Rinse in blood-heat (body temperature) water. You could use this recipe if you run out of soap. It's how cricket whites used to be cleaned.

Dealing with germs at day care

You can't avoid bugs, but you can keep their spread to a minimum. When children arrive home after day care or kindy, run a bath and add ½ teaspoon of tea tree oil to the bath water. Germs on their skin will be washed off.

Teach children how to blow their nose and cover up a cough or sneeze. The healthier your child, the less likely they are to catch a bug and become sick. Never send a child to day care if they have open wounds or a green-snot runny nose.

The best way to prevent the spread of germs is to teach your children to regularly wash their hands. They should wash before eating, after using the toilet, and after playing with animals or in a sandpit. Washing hands minimises the spread of germs.

TOY SAFETY

The Australian Competition and Consumer Commission has a 'Choke Check' to help you work out which objects might pose a hazard for children up to the age of 36 months. The Choke Check is a cylinder which mimics the size and shape of a child's throat. If an object fits completely inside the cylinder, it could get stuck in a baby's throat or be swallowed, so keep it out of their reach. Small parts of toys can easily detach and present a choking risk. Some toys designed for older children may present a choking risk for babies and toddlers. You can find the Choke Check at www.productsafety.gov.au/chokecheck.[20]

20 www.productsafety.gov.au/content/index.phtml/itemId/1007992

Top five tips for buying safe toys[21]

1. Read and follow any warning labels or safety information carefully.
2. Make sure toys are age-appropriate and check the age grading on the packaging. Toys designed for older children can be dangerous for babies.
3. Check that toys for children under the age of three don't present a choking hazard, and check that no small parts can come off.
4. Make sure any battery compartments are secure – lithium 'button' batteries can cause serious internal injuries and death if swallowed. See www.productsafety.gov.au/content/index.phtml/tag/batterycontrolled for more information.
5. Make sure there are no accessible small magnets. These can cause serious internal injuries and death if a young child swallows more than one.

 If a toy is scratchy when you hold it, roll it over your face. If it's uncomfortable on your skin, it's not safe for your baby. Babies shouldn't play with toys that have Velcro on them because the spiky plastic can scratch their skin.

 Store paints out of reach of young children. It's safer and you won't have to deal with a major clean-up if paint spills. Paint can be difficult to remove.

---

21 www.productsafety.gov.au/content/index.phtml/itemId/1007992

Children often drop small items like doll accessories or building blocks on the floor. An easy way to find them is to place either a sock or pantyhose between the head and tube of the vacuum cleaner. When you vacuum, the item will become trapped and won't go into the bag. After turning off the vacuum cleaner, remove the sock or pantyhose to find a sack of toy bits.

Problem: **Coloured pencil on hard surfaces**

What to use: **Tea tree oil, wholemeal brown bread, methylated spirits, cloth**

How to apply: Place 2 drops of tea tree oil on a slice of wholemeal brown bread (not wholegrain) and wipe over the marks. For watercolour pencils, wipe with methylated spirits on a cloth.

Problem: **Children's paint on hard surfaces**

What to use: **Water, cloth, dishwashing liquid; methylated spirits**

How to apply: Blot with water on a cloth until removed. For fresh vinyl-based paint, blot with a couple of drops of dishwashing liquid on a damp, cold cloth. For water-based paint, use methylated spirits on a cotton bud or cotton ball.

Problem: **Glitter acrylic paint on hard surfaces**

What to use: **Methylated spirits, cloth, plastic wrap, damp cloth**

How to apply: Wring a cloth in methylated spirits, place over the stain, cover the area with plastic wrap and leave for 4 hours. Remove and wipe stain with a damp cloth.

Problem: **Ballpoint pen/bottled ink (non gel) marks on hard surfaces**

What to use: **Rotten milk, cold water, bathroom soap; white spirits, cotton ball**

How to apply: Rot some full cream milk in the sun. Place the rotten milk solids over the stain. Leave until the ink is absorbed into the solids. Remove the solids with cold water. Scribble with a cake of bathroom soap run under blood-heat (body temperature) water. For red ink, wipe with white spirits on a cotton ball first.

Problem: **Fluorescent glow stick liquid on fabric**

What to use: **Uniodised salt, bucket, freezer**

How to apply: Soak the item in 1 cup of uniodised salt to a 4 litre bucket of cold water. Soak for 20 minutes. Then place in the freezer until frozen. Remove and wash according to the fabric.

Problem: **Liquid marker on hard surface or fabric**

What to use: **Methylated spirits, cotton ball; or white spirits, cotton ball, talcum powder**

How to apply: The solvent is either methylated spirits or white spirits. Test which to use by wiping with both solvents separately on a cotton bud. If marker colour comes away, that's the solvent.

Wipe the solvent in circles using a cotton ball.
You may need to use several cotton balls.
Sprinkle with talcum powder. When dry, wipe
with a damp cloth or wash according to the
fabric.

Problem: **Permanent marker**
What to use: **Same permanent marker, white spirits,**
cotton ball, talcum powder
How to apply: Permanent marker contains its own solvent so
draw over the mark with the same permanent
marker. Wipe with white spirits on a cotton
bud or cotton ball. Sprinkle with talcum
powder.

Problem: **Play dough on carpet**
What to use: **Stiff brush, vacuum cleaner, uniodised**
salt, toothbrush; or unprocessed wheat
bran, white vinegar, UV light
How to apply: Allow the play dough to dry, then scrub with
a stiff brush and vacuum as you scrub. Scrub
with a little uniodised salt on a toothbrush.
For large areas, sprinkle with unprocessed
wheat bran and scrub before vacuuming. To
remove colour, wipe with white vinegar on
a cloth and expose to sunlight or UV light.
(If using a UV light, protect areas around the
stain with cardboard.) Check every 2 hours.
Vacuum thoroughly. Repeat until removed.

Smelly teddy

Q: 'We have a much-loved old teddy bear which is starting to smell. Is there a way to make him less stinky?' asks Jane.

Problem:	**Smelly teddy bear**
What to use:	**Unprocessed wheat bran, white vinegar, oil of cloves, pillowcase**
How to apply:	Mix 1 cup of unprocessed wheat bran with drops of white vinegar until the mixture forms clumps that resemble breadcrumbs. If the teddy smells mouldy, add 2 drops of oil of cloves. Put the mixture into a pillowcase and place the smelly teddy inside. Secure the top of the pillowcase and shake well. Remove the teddy bear (preferably outside or over a bin) and brush away the bran. If the teddy bear is still smelly, find a dry-cleaner who works with conservation pieces.

DID YOU KNOW? The mandatory standard AS/NZS ISO 8124 makes it illegal to sell toys and finger paints with unsafe levels of lead and other elements in Australia. If you are concerned that toys, including antique toys, might contain lead, use a lead-testing kit available from paint stores.

Playpens

Here are some guidelines if you are buying a playpen for your child.

- Sides – at least 500 mm high
- Spaces between bars – between 50 mm and 95 mm (larger gaps can trap your baby's head)
- Folding parts should have latches that lock securely and can't be undone by your baby or toddler
- No sharp fittings or parts that can snag your baby's clothes.
- Sturdy – won't tip over when your baby leans on the sides.

How to clean a playpen

Clean a playpen by spraying with 1 teaspoon of lavender oil in a 1 litre spray pack of water. Never leave a heap of toys in the playpen, and set it up away from hazards such as blind cords, electrical appliances, furniture, etc. Keep your baby within sight when in the playpen and never leave them alone in a playpen. Make sure all latches are locked securely before use. Stop using the playpen when your baby can undo the latches. Don't use a portable cot as a playpen.

⚠ WARNING

Mobiles and toys attached to a playpen should be out of reach of kicking feet or waving hands and should be removed when your baby or toddler begins to push up on their hands and knees. They can become a choking or suffocating hazard.

TIP Don't sit babies on the kitchen floor. It's grotty and has more bacteria than other parts of the house. Place them on a bunny rug or inside a playpen.

Make your own washable toy

You'll need an old hand towel and some acrylic paint. Use the paint to draw a face on one corner of the towel. Allow it to dry. Roll the towel into a sausage and stitch it into position with heavy thread. It's easy to wash.

If making stuffed toys, use polyester filling and wrap each area of stuffing separately in pantyhose so it's easy to contain. Toddlers won't be able to chew through pantyhose to the stuffing, which can be a choking risk.

TOY BOXES

Step into most children's rooms and you're confronted by a mass of toys. The challenge is how to store them all. Shannon is a big believer in clear plastic boxes with lids. She's also a big believer in the child sorting out which toys live in which boxes. Because the container is clear, they can see what's inside. You can use cupboards for storage, but avoid stacking toys on bookshelves because when the shelves are full, the toys fall off. Don't keep large lockable containers in children's rooms in case they get stuck.

Choose toy boxes that either don't have a lid or have one that's lightweight and easily removable. Place stoppers on the inside of the lid to create a gap of 12 mm or more when the lid is closed. This stops the lid from crushing fingers and allows a trapped baby to breathe. Ensure there are ventilation holes in the lid in case a child becomes trapped inside the toy box.

How to make your own play rug

Cut an old strong sheet or a length of canvas into a large square big enough to play on. Attach a curtain ring to each corner and add 2 lengths of cotton tape to two of the rings so you can gather the four corners and tie them together. Decorate your play rug using felt-tipped pens, fabric paints or folk-art paints. You could draw a map of a town, fields, lakes, rivers or castles. Paint winding roads, a playground or an aquarium. Leave your design to completely dry and spray both sides with waterproof spray available at hardware stores.

This play rug is very portable, creates an instant play area, protects the carpet and is easy to pack up quickly: simply pick up the four rings, tie them together and you have a neat bundle that can be hung up.

How to organise toys in the bathroom

You're bound to have an array of toys in the bath. To help with cleaning, and to avoid sitting or stepping on a sharp piece of plastic, keep a toy net in the bathroom. Make your own with nylon netting available from a fabric or hardware store; it comes in a variety of colours. Attach two large stainless steel curtain rings to either end, then pull the ends together and thread through the rings with cord. Hang the toy net on a hook in the bathroom where it can drain. You could also reuse orange netting bags from the fruit market for smaller toys – especially if orange matches your bathroom.

 Take a play rug with you when travelling. You'll have somewhere clean and safe for your baby to play no matter where you are. Cart it in your nappy bag.

How to make play dough

Sift 1 cup of plain flour, ½ cup of salt and 2 tablespoons of cream of tartar into a saucepan. Gradually add 1 cup of water and 1 tablespoon of vegetable oil and stir until smooth. Add a few drops of food colouring and 2 drops of oil of cloves. Cook over a medium heat, stirring constantly for 2 minutes or until the mixture comes away from the side of the pan. Remove the pan from the heat and leave until the dough is just warm. Knead until it's soft and form it into a ball. Store in plastic wrap or inside a plastic container (the oil of cloves and salt prevent it from going mouldy).

Even though this playdough looks like a lolly, most kids won't eat it because it tastes awful. If they do like the flavour, it's non-toxic.

How to make your own children's paint

Mix ½ cup cornflour with 2 cups of water in a saucepan, bring to the boil and cook until it thickens. Allow to cool, place in an ice-cube tray and use food colourings to make different colours.

How to create a busy box

Create a busy box by collecting used paper towel rolls, egg cartons, pegs, pencils, odd bits of felt, glue, scissors, braid, scraps of fabric, wool, glitter, ribbon, feathers, cardboard and old wrapping paper. Put them all together in a box. When your children say they're bored and have nothing to do, tell them to grab the busy box and make something. Add items to it regularly so there are new things to create.

How to create a dress up box

Use old clothes of your own or from op shops and garage sales or hand-me-downs. Keep old scarves, shoes, belts, hats, ties and add them to the box. Dad's old shirts make perfect kings' coats. Make some props: spray paint a circle of paper or light cardboard gold to make a crown. Ask children to make up a story to go with their dress ups and have them act it out. Food can be organised in line with the theme they choose.

What to do with old toys

- Pass on old toys to family or friends or donate them to charity.
- Organise a toy swap party with friends and family or sell them online.
- Keep the wheels from ride-on toys to reuse.
- Keep rubberised handle covers from bike handles and use them on garden tools.
- Many old toys can be pulled apart and turned into new contraptions or inventions. Keep the parts in the kids' busy box.

CHAPTER 7

OUT AND ABOUT

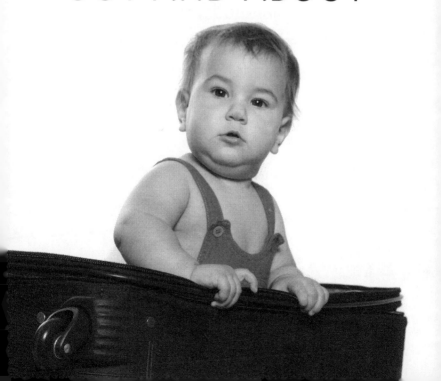

It's time to leave home and get out and about. When your baby is young, most trips will tend to be short, such as a visit to the park or to see friends. But you might find yourself taking a longer trip on a plane, particularly if relatives live overseas. By the time your children are toddlers, you'll have the routine down pat. You can avoid feeling like a loaded dromedary with some organisation and preparation.

SHORT TRIPS

Plan your trip according to how long you'll be away from home and take extra just in case – mishaps will happen. In the first 6 months, you'll generally only be away from home for a couple of hours at a time. You'll have to sort out food, clothing and transport.

Food

If your baby is under 6 months, you'll either breastfeed or use formula. If you want added privacy or if baby is easily distracted, take a protective cloth to cover the baby and your shoulder during feeding. If using formula, you have two options. If your trip is under 2 hours, you can store and transport warm formula in a thermos, but it can't be used after more than 2 hours because bacteria builds and it turns into yoghurt. If your trip is over 2 hours, keep hot water in a thermos and use it to heat the bottle. To do this, you'll need a container large enough to hold the baby bottle and the hot water.

For babies over 6 months and eating solids, the easiest food to transport is an avocado. Store a knife and spoon in a clean bag and use the knife to cut the avocado, remove the flesh and mash it with the spoon. Another easy item of food to carry is a banana – again, mash it up so it's easy to eat. If feeding fresh fruit to your child, be aware that seeds and pieces of skin can be a choking hazard. Shannon suggests placing cut fruit into the centre of a piece of boiled cotton gauze (30 cm²) and tightly tying it into a ball. The baby can suck and chew on it without risk. If taking prepared food, store it in a glass jar with a screw top lid so you can reseal it. It's common for toddlers to only eat half of the food offered, reject the rest, and say they're hungry again later on. With a screw top lid, you can store the leftovers ready for them to eat later. Another food option is homemade rusks. See p. 69 for Shannon's recipe.

Whenever there is food, there are spills and stains, so take a damp washer or wipes with you. Carry a bottle of sterilised water to use when cleaning or for the baby to sip on. If you are using baby wipes, wipe over your baby with a damp cloth afterwards, to remove the chemicals from their skin. And in case there isn't a bin nearby, keep used plastic bags in your nappy bag for rubbish. Shannon uses ecobags that break down in landfill.

Clothing

Even if you're only heading out for 2 hours, take a change of clothes and a jacket or bunny rug in case the weather changes. As a rule, dress your baby in one more layer than you're wearing – they feel changes in temperature more than you do. And don't forget to protect their heads with a hat. In summer, take a fold-up fan and ensure baby is protected from the sun. When it's hot, feed your baby twice as often as usual – it's important to keep up their fluids in the heat.

The ultimate nappy bag

There are many fantastic nappy bags to choose from. Select one that opens out so you can see everything at once – it's much easier than constantly searching for what you need. Ideally, have a bag that converts into a nappy changing mat with two solid parts that form bumpers to stop your baby from rolling. When changing your baby, place a towel on top of the mat. To clean, wipe with a damp cloth and dry in sunshine. If you get urine or poo on the mat, wipe it with white vinegar and place in sunshine.

A nappy bag should have compartments for nappies, creams and lotions. Choose a bag with a shoulder strap so you can carry the bag while keeping both hands free for the baby. Opt for a darker rather than pale-coloured bag to conceal wear and tear and stains. If taking a sheepskin, roll it up, attach it to the side of the bag and cover it with a pillowcase.

What to take in your ultimate nappy bag

- Nappies (twice as many as you think you'll need)
- Nappy cream – papaw is versatile
- Bottle of water (sterilised)
- 2 washers in zip-lock bag
- Baby soap
- Used plastic bags
- Change of clothes
- Wipes
- Spare pilchers
- Cotton gauze or mosquito net
- Food
- Sheepskin
- Fold-up umbrella – for rain and sun (with soft tips on the ribs)

- Sarong – to cover the baby or pram
- As soon as you get home, wash any dirty items in the washing machine. Don't leave them to fester in the bag.

TRANSPORT

Baby and child carriers

If walking with your baby, there are several carry options, from wraps to carriers. Wrap slings are made from one piece of fabric. You place your baby in the fabric, then wrap the sling around your body and secure it by tying the ends. Pouch slings have a sash of fabric you wear on one shoulder. The baby is placed in the pouch with the sling across the front of your body. Be careful using a sling with a baby under four months old. Young babies can't hold or turn their heads to get fresh air if needed. Follow this advice:

T – Tight: the sling should fit tightly.

I – In view at all times: your baby's face should always be in view.

C – Close enough to kiss: you should be able to reach your baby's head and kiss it.

K – Keep chin off the chest: make sure your baby can breathe.

S – Supported back: with your baby's tummy and chest against you.

There are many styles of carrier available. When choosing a carrier, consider how easy it is to put on and to put the baby in and out of, and consider the weight distribution – you don't want too much pressure on your back. When buying a carrier, take your baby with you to make sure it's a safe and comfortable fit for you both. In all cases, read and follow the manufacturer's instructions.

Prams and strollers

The pram or stroller should have a five-point restraint harness that goes around your baby's waist and between their legs. All prams and strollers should have parking brakes, with red parking brake levers. If yours isn't coloured red, wrap red tape over the lever so it's easy for you to see.

Safety tips from the ACCC

- Always read and follow the manufacturer's instructions.
- Always park the pram or stroller parallel to hazards – such as water, roads, car parks or railway tracks – so it can't roll into danger.
- Stay with your baby while they're in the pram or stroller.
- Apply the parking brake when the pram or stroller is stationary.
- Use the tether strap and harness.
- Check that frame latches and fabric fasteners are locked before use.
- Always watch your baby while they are in the pram or stroller.
- Only use the pram or stroller for the intended number of babies.

- Stop your baby from standing in or leaning out of the pram or stroller.
- Watch other children and stop them from climbing into or leaning on the pram or stroller.
- Remove your baby from the pram or stroller before adjusting any moving parts.
- Supervise other children outside the pram or stroller and keep children and fingers away from the hinge mechanism when folding and unfolding the pram or stroller.
- Never use a pram or stroller as a substitute for a cot. If your baby is left to sleep in a pram or stroller, they can become trapped between parts and strangle or suffocate.
- Never use a pillow, cushion or bumpers in a pram or stroller.
- Never hang shopping bags on handles, as these can tip the pram or stroller over.
- Don't let other young children push the pram or stroller without your help.
- Supervise your baby if they fall asleep in the pram. It's not designed to sleep in.

⚠ WARNING

When setting up your pram, use two hands. Don't set it up juggling your baby on your hip – it's not safe.

 If trying to get your baby to sleep in the pram, roll it over rough ground. The vibration helps send them to sleep.

Problem: **Dirty pram**

What to use: **Dishwashing liquid, spray pack, brush, cloth, sunshine; uniodised salt, oil of cloves, bucket, nylon brush; damp tea bag, pantyhose**

How to apply: To clean plastic, mix 1 teaspoon of dishwashing liquid with 1 litre of water in a spray pack. Spray the mixture over the pram and scrub with a brush. Rinse with a damp cloth and dry in sunshine. To clean canvas, dissolve 1 kilo of uniodised salt and ¼ teaspoon of oil of cloves in a 9 litre bucket of water. Scrub with the mixture using a nylon brush. Leave in the sun until dry, then brush the salt off. To clean aluminium, wipe with a damp tea bag in the toe of pantyhose.

TIP To clean stroller wheels, place a dampened polypropylene fibre mat (available at pet stores) at the entrance to your home and run the wheels over it, then run the wheels over a dry mat. The less dirt you bring inside your house, the less cleaning you'll have to do.

Mouldy stroller

Q: 'I left the stroller in the boot of the car and it's now mouldy,' says Murray. 'Can it be fixed?'

Problem:	Mouldy stroller
What to use:	Uniodised salt, bucket, warm water, stiff broom, oil of cloves
How to apply:	Dissolve 1 kilo of uniodised salt in a 9 litre bucket of warm water and apply to the stroller. Leave it to dry with the salt coating. Then remove the salt with a stiff broom and the mould will come off with it. To prevent more mould, add 2 drops of oil of cloves to the water.

How to choose a travel cot or portacot

Choose a travel cot with removable fabric that clips into position. The fabric can be removed and washed in the washing machine. Avoid travel cots with unlined mesh because babies can rip their nails in the nylon meshing.

Outings to the pool or beach

Most babies and toddlers love being in water. There's even a phrase for it – 'water baby'. One thing to watch when swimming with your baby is their temperature – they feel the cold more easily than adults. If they start shivering, remove them from the water and warm them in a dry towel. Also, chlorine used in pools can be harsh on little lungs, so if there's a strong chlorine smell, leave the pool. Be careful with sun exposure and be aware that no sunscreen can offer 100 per cent protection from the sun. Keep babies in the shade, especially between 10 am and 3 pm.

What to do if there's a 'poonami' – a poo explosion

Blow outs are common and are never fun, especially the down-the-leg, up-the-back ones. If a 'poonami' happens away from home, get to the nearest toilet or changing room (if you can), grab a plastic bag from your nappy bag, wrap the plastic bag over your hand so it's covered entirely and catch the bulk of the poo in the plastic bag. Remove, tie up and dispose of in a bin. Wipe as much poo from your baby or toddler as you can (using a washer and water or wipes), then put on a new nappy and spare set of clothes. If there's no changing room, after catching as much poo as possible in the plastic bag and using the washer and water or wipes, place the dirty clothing in another plastic bag to deal with when you get home. When you get home, wash your baby in the bath. To clean post-poonami clothing, soak items overnight in cold water with ¼ cup of bicarb, then wash in the washing machine and hang in sunshine. Remember: the water needs to be cold because it's a protein stain. Sunshine will fade any remaining marks.

Essential pool/beach bag

- Waterproof pool/beach bag
- Swim nappies (these are not leakproof, so you'll need to change them quickly to avoid leakage in the pool), regular nappy, dry change of clothes
- Sunscreen – water resistant broad spectrum designed for toddlers or for sensitive skin. Reapply every 2 hours.

- Plastic bag for wet gear and towels
- With toddlers, take snacks. In a cooler bag with ice, have fruit, yoghurt, sandwiches and dips.
- ¼ teaspoon of tea tree oil with 1 litre of water in a spray pack (to use in the changing room)

Problem:	**Dirty swimming costume**
What to use:	**White vinegar, bucket**
How to apply:	Never wash with laundry detergent, which breaks down latex and elastane, making swimmers perish, pucker and lose elasticity. To clean, rinse in 1 cup of white vinegar per 9 litre bucket of water. If you rinse right after swimming, the swimming costume will last longer. Dry in sunshine.

 When you're out, have a technique to get your children's attention in case of danger. One suggestion is that when you say 'hands behind backs', they have to stop still with their hands behind their backs until you instruct them to move again.

CAR

Shannon bans everyone from eating and drinking in the car. She reckons if your child can hold their own food, they're old enough to wait until the end of the journey before eating. You'll be using your boot to carry the pram and other gear, so clean it out before baby arrives. If the boot floor is covered in oil or dirt, place an old sheet over it. Don't store a stroller on the back seat of the car because it's dangerous. A sudden stop could cause it to fly. If you need to change a nappy in the car, put a change mat down first – cleaning car upholstery isn't easy.

Baby car seat and capsules

As mentioned before, many people hire capsules because you only use them for about 6 months. If hiring one, even if it looks clean, wipe it with a cloth sprayed with ¼ teaspoon of tea tree oil in 1 litre of water in a spray pack and place it in sunshine. It's important the restraint fits snugly with no slack or twisted straps. At the end of your trip, take your baby or toddler out of the car seat or capsule even if it means waking them; it's not safe for young children to spend long periods of time in booster seats, infant seats or capsules. For added safety, place webbing or a fold-up dome over the capsule in case of an accident. Clean in the same way as a pram.

 Cut back on cleaning your child's car seat by using a car seat liner. Make your own with a cotton pillowcase wrapped over the entire chair and cut where the straps come through.

How to choose a car seat

When it's time for a baby seat, choose one with a five-point harness – you don't want toddlers to be able to wriggle out. Keep straps clean and remove food, spit and gunk promptly.

Problem: **Dirty car seat/upholstery**
What to use: **Dishwashing liquid, water, cloth, sunshine, vacuum cleaner, lemon juice**
How to apply: Remove the car seat from the car and shake off debris. Mix ½ teaspoon of dishwashing liquid in 1 litre of water to generate a frothy mix. Wipe with the froth on a cloth. Rinse with a damp cloth and dry in sunshine. When dry, vacuum. Wipe with lemon juice to remove the smell.

Problem: **Dirty baby capsule**
What to use: **Uniodised salt, bucket, water, cloth, oil of cloves**
How to apply: Wipe with 1 kilo of uniodised salt mixed in a 9 litre bucket of water and rinse thoroughly. Wipe over the edges with a cloth sprayed with ¼ teaspoon oil of cloves in a 1 litre bottle of water – babies often suck on the edges. Baby spit is a combination of milk and moisture – an ideal environment for mould to grow.

Problem: **Vomit in the car**
What to use: **Cloth, bicarb, vacuum cleaner, glycerine; or cake of bathroom soap, cloth, lemon juice**
How to apply: If you can, remove the seat from the car, wipe away the vomit with a damp cloth, sprinkle with bicarb and place in the sun. When

dry, vacuum. Clean plastics with glycerine applied with a cloth. If the vomit is on the upholstery of the car, remove as much vomit as possible with a damp cloth, then scribble the upholstery with a cake of bathroom soap and cold water, remove the soap with a damp cloth, and allow to dry. Wipe with lemon juice to remove the smell.

TAKING YOUR BABY ON PUBLIC TRANSPORT

If you're using a pram, trains are easier to get on and off than buses because there's a larger access area in the carriage. This assumes there's a lift at the railway station. When catching a bus, take your baby out of the pram and hold them. Prams don't have a wide wheelbase compared with their height and are likely to topple over. Any unusual movement can send them flying.

For obvious reasons, avoid travelling during peak hour. Plan your trip before you go – use online services for timetables and amenities such as lifts at railway stations and transport interchanges.

PLANE TRAVEL

You'll need to be very organised for this task. When booking the flight, ask if you can reserve the bulkhead seat – or at least an aisle seat. Never choose a window seat with a baby, unless you are with family or friends because you'll be climbing over other travellers, under 2 years generally sit on your lap with an extension seat belt. On most long haul flights, carrycots are available. If you've booked a separate seat, most airlines allow you to bring a car seat for babies over 6 months but under 18 kilograms to sit in. Check with the airline first.

Feed babies regularly during the flight, especially during take off and landing because the sucking action helps to equalise pressure in their ears. When they are older, give them barley sugar to suck on so their ears pop. Another option is to place your mouth over your baby's nose and give a light puff of air – this makes them cough. They don't know how to yawn. If your child has ear pain, soak a paper towel in hot water, put the towel in the bottom of a cup and hold the cup against their ear.

The best age to take a baby on a plane is between 3 and 9 months. After 9 months, they're more mobile and travel is a greater challenge.

Some airlines provide a limited range of baby food, milk, baby bottles, cereals and rusks but it's a good idea to take on board food and drink your baby is used to. Keep your child hydrated during the flight, particularly on longer flights, to counteract the dry air on board.

Some airlines allow you to carry a reasonable quantity of liquid, aerosol or gel products for a baby or toddler for the duration of the flight and any delays that might occur. A 'reasonable quantity' is at the discretion of security screening officers at customs.

Baby products may include:

- baby milk, including breast milk
- sterilised water
- juice
- baby food in liquid, gel or paste form
- disposable wipes.

Baby milk powder (not liquid) and gels can be taken onboard. Most airlines will warm a bottle for you, but not all provide this service so check beforehand. If the airline doesn't warm milk, start giving your baby cold milk a few weeks before flying so they get used to it. Place baby food, yoghurt, cheese and puddings in 100 ml containers and store in clear plastic bags.

Have a well-stocked nappy bag to take onboard. For international flights, make sure all liquids and gels are under 100 ml. Any medication you want to take on board that's not prescription medication also has to be under 100 ml and kept in a clear plastic bag. For toddlers, make sure you have plenty of snacks. Depending on how long the flight is, pack two or three changes of clothes in case there are spills and stains.

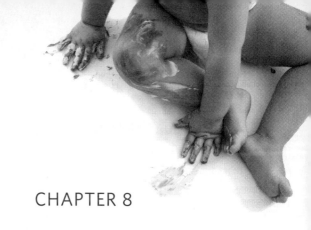

CHAPTER 8

A–Z
STAIN REMOVAL

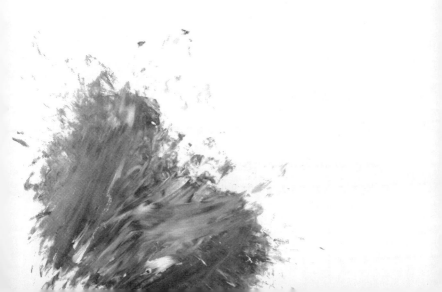

APPLE JUICE

On carpet/upholstery

- Remove excess by blotting with paper towel.
- Brush across the surface with 2 drops of glycerine on a toothbrush (don't push it into the backing). Leave for 90 minutes.
- Tightly wring a cloth in white vinegar and wipe out the glycerine.
- Sprinkle with talcum powder.
- When dry, vacuum. If there's still a tannin mark after 24 hours, repeat.

On cotton/fabric

- Remove excess under the tap using blood-heat (body temperature) water.
- Rub with 2 drops of glycerine. Leave for 90 minutes.
- Wash according to the fabric. If the stain has disappeared, dry in sunshine. If not, repeat.

AVOCADO

This is high in fat and can leave a greasy mark.

On carpet/upholstery

- Remove excess by lifting with a plastic comb or blotting with paper towel.

- Massage with a couple of drops of dishwashing liquid on your fingertips until the liquid feels like jelly.
- Rub with a damp pair of loosely rolled pantyhose.
- Wipe with a damp cloth until the dishwashing liquid is removed.
- Absorb moisture by covering the area with paper towel. Place a book on top of the paper towel to assist with absorption.

On cotton/fabric

- Remove excess under the tap using blood-heat (body temperature) water.
- Massage with a couple of drops of dishwashing liquid on your fingertips until the liquid feels like jelly.
- Rinse using blood-heat water.
- Wash according to the fabric. Dry on the clothesline or clothes airer.

BABY BOTTLES

To clean

- Rinse bottles with cold water first until no milk remains (hot water sets proteins). Rinse bottles as soon after feeding as possible.
- Wash in the sink in warm water and a little dishwashing liquid. Use a bottle brush to clean the inside of bottles.
- Rinse in clean water. Then sterilise.

To sterilise

- Fill a large pot with water and add 2 tablespoons of salt. Bring to the boil.
- Place bottles and teats in the pot.
- Turn off the heat and leave for 10 minutes.
- Rinse the bottles in boiled water (hot or cold) to remove residual salt. Allow to air dry.
- If you can, avoid using the dishwasher because of detergent residue. Once your baby is over 6 months (9 months if formula fed), use the dishwasher but replace the detergent with bicarb (in the wash slot) and white vinegar (in the rinse slot).

BABY FOOD

Removing baby food stains depends on what's in the food. It could contain carbohydrates, proteins, or natural pigments from fruit and vegetables. Consult the relevant technique.

BABY FORMULA

This is harder to remove than breast milk because it contains complex enzymes. When feeding, have a cloth nearby to wipe away any spills.

On carpet/upholstery

- Remove excess by lifting with a plastic comb or by blotting with paper towel.

- Scribble with a cake of bathroom soap run under cold water.
- Scrub with a toothbrush in every direction – north, south, east and west.
- If the stain is older than 1 hour, wipe with 2 drops of glycerine on a toothbrush in every direction (don't push it into the backing). Leave for 90 minutes. Then scribble with a cake of bathroom soap.
- Wipe with a damp cloth.
- Absorb moisture by covering the area with paper towel. Place a book on top of the paper towel to assist with absorption.

On cotton/fabric (not wool)

- Remove excess under the tap using cold water.
- Scribble with a cake of bathroom soap. Rub the fabric against itself using your hands.
- If the stain is older than 1 hour, brush across the surface with 2 drops of glycerine on a toothbrush. Leave for 90 minutes. Then scribble with bathroom soap.
- Rinse using cold water.
- Wash according to the fabric. Dry on the clothesline or clothes airer.

On wool

- Remove excess under the tap using cold water.
- Scribble with a cake of bathroom soap. Gently rub the wool against itself using your hands.
- Wash the entire garment straightaway in 1 teaspoon of cheap shampoo and blood-heat (body temperature) water.

- Rinse in blood-heat water.
- Gently wring and dry flat on a towel in the shade.

BABY OIL

On carpet/upholstery

- Remove excess by blotting with paper towel.
- Massage the stain with a couple of drops of dishwashing liquid (undiluted) on your fingertips until the liquid feels like jelly.
- Wipe with a damp cloth until the dishwashing liquid is removed.
- Absorb moisture by covering the area with paper towel. Place a book on top of the paper towel to assist with absorption.

On cotton/fabric

- Massage the stain with a couple of drops of dishwashing liquid (undiluted) on your fingertips until the liquid feels like jelly.
- Rinse using blood-heat (body temperature) water.
- Wash according to the fabric. Dry on the clothesline or clothes airer.

 To clean several items covered in baby oil, such as towels, place them in a big bucket filled with blood-heat (body temperature) water and dishwashing liquid and stomp on them with your feet. It's easiest to do in the shower. Then empty the items into the washing machine and wash straightaway or the oil will reset.

BANANA

On carpet/upholstery

- Remove excess by lifting with a plastic comb or by blotting with paper towel.
- Brush across the surface with 2 drops of glycerine on a toothbrush (don't push it into the backing). Leave for 90 minutes.
- Tightly wring a cloth in white vinegar and wipe out the glycerine.
- Sprinkle with talcum powder.
- When dry, vacuum. If there's still a tannin mark after 24 hours, repeat.
- Alternatively, mix *Vanish NapiSan Oxi Action Sensitive Powder* and water to form a paste the consistency of spreadable butter and place on the stain for a few minutes.
- Wipe with a damp cloth.
- Absorb moisture by covering the area with paper towel. Place a book on top of the paper towel to assist with absorption.
- When dry, vacuum.

On cotton/fabric

- Remove excess under the tap using cold water.
- Wipe with 2 drops of glycerine on a cloth.
- Wash according to the fabric. Dry on the clothesline or clothes airer.

On granite/marble/stone

- Remove excess by lifting with a plastic comb or by blotting with paper towel.
- Mix plaster of Paris and water to the consistency of peanut butter.
- To each cup of mixture, add 1 teaspoon of glycerine.
- Spread 5 mm to 1 cm thick over the stain.
- Allow to dry completely. If it feels cold on the back of your hand, it's not dry.
- When dry, brush off.

 TIP To remove stains caused by banana seeds – the black bits inside a banana – wipe with glycerine, leave for 90 minutes and wash normally. If you've already washed the item, mix equal parts glycerine and tea tree oil and place over the stain for 90 minutes, then wash again. It's unlikely, but if there's staining from banana sap, wipe with glycerine, then wipe with white spirits on a cotton ball.

BERRY

When removing berry stains, don't use soap or heat because it will set the stain.

On carpet/upholstery

- Remove excess by lifting with a plastic comb or by blotting with paper towel.

- For berry stains that change colour (blueberry, blackberry), wipe with 2 drops of glycerine on a cloth. Leave for 5 minutes. Then tightly wring a cloth in white vinegar so it's damp but not wet. Blot over the mark. Place the vinegar cloth in one hand and a dry cloth in the other and wipe hand over hand, as though stroking a cat, until the stain is removed.
- For other berries (strawberry, raspberry, etc.), tightly wring a cloth in white vinegar so it's damp but not wet. Blot over the mark.
- Absorb moisture by covering the area with paper towel. Place a book on top of the paper towel to assist with absorption.

On cotton/fabric (not silk/wool)

- Remove excess under the tap using cold water.
- For berry stains that change colour (blueberry, blackberry), wipe with 2 drops of glycerine on a cloth. Then tightly wring a cloth in white vinegar and blot over the mark.
- For other berries (strawberry, raspberry, etc.), tightly wring a cloth in white vinegar and blot over the mark.
- In all cases, wash according to the fabric. Dry in sunshine.

On silk/wool

- Blot with white vinegar on a cloth until the berry colour is removed.
- Massage with 1 teaspoon of cheap shampoo on your fingertips.
- Rinse in blood-heat (body temperature) water.

- Rinse in 1 teaspoon of cheap hair conditioner and blood-heat water.
- Gently wring and dry flat on a towel in the shade. Ensure silk is dried away from the wind so the fibres don't tangle and leave a dusty look.

BETADINE

On carpet/upholstery

- Remove excess by blotting with paper towel.
- Massage with 2 drops of lavender oil on a cloth. Tightly wring a cloth in white vinegar so it's damp but not wet. Blot over the mark.
- Alternatively, remove excess then scrub with 2 drops of glycerine on a toothbrush in all directions – north, south, east and west. For an old stain, leave overnight. Rub with a little dishwashing liquid on a cloth. Wipe with a damp cloth until the dishwashing liquid is removed. Tightly wring a cloth in white vinegar, fold the cloth flat and polish out the glycerine without pushing it into the back of the carpet or upholstery.
- In both cases, absorb moisture by covering the area with paper towel. Place a book on top of the paper towel to assist with absorption.

On cotton/fabric

- Massage with 2 drops of lavender oil on a cloth.
- Wash according to the fabric. Dry on the clothesline or clothes airer.

On stone

- Sprinkle with talcum powder like icing sugar on a cake.
- Spray with white vinegar. Leave for 15 minutes.
- Scrub with 2 drops of lavender oil on a brush.

BLACKCURRANT JUICE (RIBENA)

This is high in vitamin C and creates a strong tannin stain.

On carpet/upholstery

- Remove excess by blotting with paper towel.
- Place 2 drops of glycerine on a toothbrush and lightly brush across the surface – don't push into the backing of the carpet or upholstery. Leave for 90 minutes.
- Tightly wring a cloth in white vinegar and wipe out the glycerine.
- Sprinkle with talcum powder.
- When dry, vacuum. If there's still a tannin mark, repeat after 24 hours.

On cotton/fabric

- Remove excess under the tap using blood-heat (body temperature) water.
- Rub with 2 drops of glycerine. Leave for 90 minutes.
- Wash according to the fabric. If the stain has disappeared, dry in sunshine. If not, repeat.

Add tea tree oil to the washing detergent when cleaning baby clothes in the washing machine. It kills bacteria and is an anti-fungal, and helps to reduce nappy rash. Never apply directly to the skin.

BLANKET

To clean

- For wool, mohair and silk, wash with 1 teaspoon of cheap shampoo in 9 litres of blood-heat (body temperature) water.
- Rinse with 1 teaspoon of cheap hair conditioner in 9 litres of blood-heat water.
- For polar fleece, acrylic and cotton, wash in the washing machine with laundry detergent.
- Dry on the clothesline pegged between two lines in a U shape. Place a sheet over the top to protect the fibres from the sun.

BLOOD

This is a protein stain so use only cold water.

On carpet/upholstery

- If you've already used a product to try to remove the blood, neutralise by blotting with white vinegar on a cloth. Scrub with 2 drops of glycerine on a toothbrush and leave for 90 minutes. Then follow the instructions below.
- Remove as much as possible by blotting with paper towel.

- Scribble over stain with a cake of bathroom soap run under cold water.
- Scrub with a toothbrush in every direction – north, south, east and west.
- Wipe with a cold damp cloth.
- Absorb moisture by covering the area with paper towel. Place a book on top of the paper towel to assist with absorption.

On cotton/fabric (not silk/wool)

- Quickly pour a large quantity of cold water through the stain.
- Scribble with a cake of bathroom soap. Rub the fabric against itself using your hands.
- If there's a shadow mark, soak in ½ lid *Vanish NapiSan Oxi Action Sensitive Powder* and 9 litres of cold water for 30 minutes. Don't use on silk or wool.
- If the stain has set, wipe with 2 drops of glycerine on a cotton ball.
- In all cases, wash according to the fabric. Dry on the clothesline or clothes airer.

On mattress

- For a fresh stain, scribble with a cake of bathroom soap run under cold water.
- Wipe with a damp cloth.
- Leave to dry. Repeat if needed.
- For an old stain, mix equal parts cornflour, glycerine and water to the consistency of thickened cream.

- Leave on the stain until it dries.
- Brush off with a stiff brush.
- You may need to repeat these steps a few times because old stains can be particularly difficult to remove.

On silk/wool

- Scribble with a cake of bathroom soap run under cold water.
- Wash in 1 teaspoon of cheap shampoo and blood-heat (body temperature) water.
- Gently wring and dry flat on a towel in the shade. Ensure silk is dried away from the wind so the fibres don't tangle and leave a dusty look.

BOTTLES/TEATS

(see BABY BOTTLES)

 TIP Store boiled water in a sterile container in the fridge. It will come in handy.

BREAST MILK

This is high in protein and sugars, so use cold water to remove. Unlike other proteins, breast milk contains its own emulsifiers. Wash in the washing machine using cold water. The best way to remove bacteria is by drying in sunshine.

On carpet/upholstery

- Remove excess by blotting with paper towel.
- Scribble with a cake of bathroom soap run under cold water.
- Wipe with a damp cloth.
- Absorb moisture by covering the area with paper towel. Place a book on top of the paper towel to assist with absorption.

On cotton/fabric

- Remove excess under the tap using cold water.
- Scribble with a cake of bathroom soap. Rub the fabric against itself using your hands.
- Rinse using cold water.
- Wash in cold water. Dry on the clothesline or clothes airer.

On wool

- Scribble with a cake of bathroom soap dipped in cold water.
- Gently rub the wool against itself using your hands.
- Wash straightaway in 1 teaspoon of cheap shampoo and blood-heat (body temperature) water. Rinse in blood-heat water.
- Gently wring and dry flat on a towel in the shade.

(see also SPIT-UP MILK)

BREAST PUMP (ELECTRIC)

To clean

- Remove parts that come into contact with breast milk.
- Rinse with cold water after pumping.
- Boil water in a pot, turn off heat and add pump parts. Leave for 10 minutes.
- Allow to dry.

CALOMINE LOTION

On carpet/upholstery

- Absorb excess with paper towel.
- Rub with a couple of drops of dishwashing liquid on your fingers until it feels like jelly.
- Wipe with a damp cloth.
- Repeat or you'll have a milky residue.
- When dry, vacuum.

On cotton/fabric

- Remove excess under the tap using cold water.
- Rub with a couple of drops of dishwashing liquid on your fingers until it feels like jelly.
- Wash according to the fabric. Dry on the clothesline or clothes airer in sunshine.

TIP If your child eats chilli that's too hot for them, give them a slice of lemon or orange to suck. The acid cuts the alkaline in chilli.

CAPSULE

To clean

- Wipe the exterior, including the handles, with a cake of bathroom soap and water.
- Alternatively, wipe with 1 cup of uniodised salt mixed in a 9 litre bucket of water.
- Wipe over the edges with a cloth sprayed with ¼ teaspoon oil of cloves in a 1 litre spray pack of water – babies often suck on the edges.
- Most baby capsules have a lining that can be removed and washed in the washing machine. It's best to use liners made of cotton.

CARROT

On carpet/upholstery

- Remove excess by lifting with a plastic comb or by blotting with paper towel.
- Tightly wring a cloth in white vinegar so it's damp but not wet. Blot over the mark.
- To remove an orange stain, expose to sunlight or UV light. (If using UV light, protect areas around the stain with cardboard.) Check every 2 hours.

- Absorb moisture by covering the area with paper towel. Place a book on top of the paper towel to assist with absorption.

On cotton/fabric (not wool)

- Remove excess under the tap using cold water.
- Blot with or soak in white vinegar until the stain is removed.
- Wash according to the fabric. Dry in sunshine.

On wool

- Place equal parts white vinegar and cold water on a cloth and wring tightly so it's damp but not wet. Blot over the mark.
- If the stain has set, wipe with 2 drops of lavender oil on a cloth. Leave for 20 minutes.
- Wash in 1 teaspoon of cheap shampoo and blood-heat (body temperature) water.
- Rinse in blood-heat water.
- Gently wring and dry flat on a towel in the shade.

CAR SEAT

Cut back on cleaning by using a car seat liner. Make your own with a cotton pillowcase wrapped over the entire chair and cut where the seat belt comes through.

To clean

- Remove the car seat from the car and shake off debris.
- Mix ½ teaspoon of dishwashing liquid in 1 litre of water.

- Wipe with the froth only on a cloth.
- Rinse with a damp cloth and dry in sunshine.
- When dry, vacuum. Wipe with lemon juice to remove smells.

CEREAL

On carpet/upholstery

- Remove excess by lifting with a plastic comb or by blotting with paper towel.
- Scribble with a cake of bathroom soap run under blood-heat (body temperature) water.
- Wipe with a damp cloth.
- Absorb moisture by covering the area with paper towel. Place a book on top of the paper towel to assist with absorption.

On cotton/fabric

- Remove excess under the tap using cold water.
- Scribble with a cake of bathroom soap. Rub the fabric against itself using your hands.
- Wash according to the fabric. Dry on the clothesline or clothes airer.

CHALK

On carpet/upholstery

- Wipe with a slice of wholemeal brown bread (not wholegrain).

- If this doesn't work, mix ½ teaspoon of dishwashing liquid with 1 cup of water and wipe onto the chalk mark with a cloth.
- Tightly wring a cloth in white vinegar so it's damp but not wet. Blot over the mark.
- Absorb moisture by covering the area with paper towel. Place a book on top of the paper towel to assist with absorption.
- Alternatively, wipe with white spirits on a cloth. Sprinkle with talcum powder.
- When dry, vacuum.

On cotton/fabric

- Remove excess under the tap using cold water.
- Scribble with a cake of bathroom soap. Rub the fabric against itself using your hands.
- Wash according to the fabric. Dry on the clothesline or clothes airer.

COLOURED PENCIL

On carpet/upholstery

- Place 2 drops of tea tree oil on a slice of wholemeal brown bread (not wholegrain) and wipe over the marks.
- Wipe with methylated spirits on a cotton bud until the colour bleeds.
- Cover with talcum powder.
- When it dries, vacuum. Repeat, if needed.

On walls

- Place 2 drops of tea tree oil on a slice of wholemeal brown bread (not wholegrain) and wipe over the marks.
- Wipe with methylated spirits on a cloth.

CORDIAL (FRUIT)

On carpet/upholstery

- Remove excess by blotting with paper towel.
- Tightly wring a cloth in white vinegar so it's damp but not wet. Blot over the mark.
- For an old stain, wipe with 2 drops of glycerine on a cloth. Leave for 90 minutes. Then blot with white vinegar on a cloth.
- For remaining coloured stains, expose to sunlight or UV light. (If using UV light, protect areas around the stain with cardboard.) Check every 2 hours.
- In all cases, absorb moisture by covering the area with paper towel. Place a book on top of the paper towel to assist with absorption.

On cotton/fabric

- Remove excess under the tap using cold water.
- Blot with or soak in white vinegar. Hang in the sunshine until the stain fades.
- Wash according to the fabric. Dry on the clothesline or clothes airer.

COT

To clean

- Wipe over hard surfaces with a cloth sprayed with ¼ teaspoon of tea tree oil in 1 litre of water in a spray pack, or with 1 teaspoon of lavender oil in 1 litre of water in a spray pack. Have one cloth covered with spray, and another dry cloth; wipe with one, then dry with the other.
- Air the mattress in sunshine.

COUGH SYRUP

Cough syrup is high in sugar. And *Children's Panadol (Cherry Vanilla Flavour)* can stain and leave marks on nappies.

On carpet/upholstery

- Remove excess by blotting with paper towel.
- Mix equal parts white vinegar and blood-heat (body temperature) water.
- Scrub the mixture with a toothbrush or pantyhose in all directions – north, south, east and west.
- Absorb moisture by covering the area with paper towel. Place a book on top of the paper towel to assist with absorption.
- When almost dry, repeat.
- To remove colouring, follow the instructions above, then expose to sunlight or UV light. (If using UV light, protect areas around the stain with cardboard.) Check every 2 hours.
- If a shadow returns in a couple of weeks, repeat.

On cotton/fabric

- Remove excess under the tap using cold water.
- Blot with or soak in white vinegar.
- If there's residue, scrub with 2 drops of glycerine on a toothbrush. Leave for 90 minutes. Blot with white vinegar and hang in sunshine until the stain fades before washing.
- Wash according to the fabric. Dry on the clothesline or clothes airer.

CREAMS

(see OINTMENT)

CRÊPE PAPER

On carpet/upholstery

- Remove excess by blotting with paper towel.
- Mix 2 drops of lavender oil and 2 drops of glycerine to form a paste.
- Apply the mixture with a cloth. Leave for 2 minutes.
- Remove with a damp cloth.
- Absorb moisture by covering the area with paper towel. Place a book on top of the paper towel to assist with absorption.

On cotton/fabric

- Mix 2 drops of lavender oil and 2 drops of glycerine to form a paste.
- Place over the item for 90 minutes.

■ Wash according to the fabric. Dry on the clothesline or clothes airer.

CUSTARD

On carpet/upholstery

■ Remove excess by lifting with a plastic comb or by blotting with paper towel.

■ Scribble with a cake of bathroom soap run under cold water.

■ Wipe with a damp cloth.

■ Massage with a couple of drops of dishwashing liquid on your fingertips until the liquid feels like jelly.

■ Wipe with a damp cloth until the dishwashing liquid is removed.

■ Absorb moisture by covering the area with paper towel. Place a book on top of the paper towel to assist with absorption.

On cotton/fabric

■ Remove excess under the tap using cold water.

■ Scribble with a cake of bathroom soap. Rub the fabric against itself using your hands. For residue, massage with a couple of drops of dishwashing liquid on your fingertips until the liquid feels like jelly.

■ Alternatively, make a paste of *Vanish NapiSan Oxi Action Sensitive Powder* and water to the consistency of spreadable butter and place over the stain. Leave for 20 minutes. Don't use on wool, silk or leather.

- In both cases, wash according to the fabric. Dry on the clothesline or clothes airer.

CRAYON

On walls/hard surfaces

- Rub over the mark with a pencil eraser damped in soapy water. The wax in the crayon will come off in balls.
- If stubborn, wipe over with bicarb on a damp cotton bud or old toothbrush (for a larger area). Don't wipe outside the crayon mark or the wall could become shiny.

DIARRHOEA

On carpet/upholstery

- Remove excess by lifting with a plastic comb or by blotting with paper towel.
- Scribble with a cake of bathroom soap run under cold water.
- Wipe with a damp cloth.
- Massage with a couple of drops of dishwashing liquid on your fingertips until the liquid feels like jelly.
- Wipe with a damp cloth until the dishwashing liquid is removed.
- Absorb moisture by covering the area with paper towel. Place a book on top of the paper towel to assist with absorption.

On cotton/fabric

- Remove excess under the tap using cold water.
- Scribble with a cake of bathroom soap run under cold water.
- Massage with a couple of drops of dishwashing liquid on your fingertips until the liquid feels like jelly.
- Rinse using cold water.
- Alternatively, mix ½ lid of *Vanish NapiSan Oxi Action Sensitive Powder* in a 9 litre bucket of cold water and soak for 20 minutes, or soak overnight in a bucket of cold water with ¼ cup of bicarb.
- In all cases, wash according to the fabric. Dry in sunshine.

DUMMIES/PACIFIERS

To clean

- Fill a large pot with water and add 2 tablespoons of salt. Bring to the boil.
- Place dummies in the pot.
- Turn off the heat and leave for 10 minutes.
- Rinse in boiled water (hot or cold) to remove residual salt. Allow to air dry.
- Alternatively, wash in hot soapy water and rinse in boiled water. Allow to air dry.

FAECES

(see POO)

FRUIT JUICE

(see JUICE)

GENTIAN VIOLET

On carpet/upholstery

- Wring a cloth in 3 per cent hydrogen peroxide and press only over the stain until it comes away.
- Wipe excess with a dry cloth, hand over hand, until removed.

On cotton/fabric

- Wipe with 3 per cent hydrogen peroxide until the stain is removed and rinse immediately.
- Wash according to the fabric. Dry on the clothesline or clothes airer.

On baby skin

- Wipe with petroleum jelly or papaw cream on a cloth. Most will come away immediately, but residue may remain. Sunshine will fade it from skin.

GLITTER

On carpet/upholstery

- Vacuum as much glitter as possible.
- Cut a cake of bathroom soap in half lengthways and round the edges. Dampen it in water and use it like a rolling pin

across the glitter. The glitter will stick to the soap. Clear the glitter from the soap under water as you go.

- Alternatively, vacuum excess, then put on rubber gloves and wash your gloved hands with a cake of bathroom soap and water. Shake your hands dry. When dry, wipe over the glitter. It will stick to the rubber.
- In both cases, absorb moisture by covering the area with paper towel. Place a book on top of the paper towel to assist with absorption.
- For glitter acrylic paint, wring a cloth in methylated spirits, place over the stain, cover the area with plastic wrap and leave for 4 hours. Remove and wipe the stain with a damp cloth.

On cotton/fabric

- Place the item on a clean towel and lightly spray over the glitter with hairspray.
- Leave until the hairspray goes hard.
- Cut a cake of bathroom soap in half lengthways and round the edges to create a soap sausage. Dampen it in water and use it like a rolling pin across the glitter. The glitter will stick to the soap. Clear the glitter from the soap under water as you go.
- Wash according to the fabric. Dry on the clothesline or clothes airer.
- For glitter acrylic paint, soak in methylated spirits for 4 hours. Then wash according to the fabric. Dry on the clothesline or clothes airer.

GLUE

Different glues have different solvents.

- Super glue – remove with super glue remover or acetone.
- Craft and PVA glues (which go on white and dry clear) – use steam.
- Two-part epoxy glues (e.g. *Araldite*) – remove with acetone.
- Gums and paper glues – wipe with a damp cloth.
- Children's craft glue – use blood-heat (body temperature) water and a cake of bathroom soap and scribble over the stain.
- Contact adhesives – remove with tea tree oil.

On carpet

- Wrap a fine-toothed metal comb in a tissue so the teeth poke through the tissue. Don't use a plastic comb.
- Place the comb at an angle to the carpet and wedge it underneath the glue.
- Dip a cotton ball in the appropriate solvent and rub over the top of the stain with the comb underneath. Use extra cotton balls, if needed. Replace the tissue if it gets wet.
- For an epoxy glue stain, warm with a hair dryer after wedging the comb underneath.
- Wring a cloth in boiling water and place it over the glue until the cloth cools.
- Pinch and pull the cloth to remove as much of the adhesive as possible.

- Repeat a few times before using the solvent.
- To remove the smell of acetone, wipe with equal parts methylated spirits and water on a cloth.

On timber

- Dampen pantyhose with water and heat in the microwave for 10 seconds – no longer or the pantyhose will melt.
- Rub over the glue in the direction of the grain using speed, not pressure.
- Dry thoroughly with a cloth.

On tulle

- Boil the kettle to generate steam.
- Hold the affected area over the steam for 1 minute.
- Rub over the glue with pantyhose. The glue will be pulled off.

On walls

- Place a drop of tea tree oil on the glue patch and cover with plastic wrap.
- Leave for 20 minutes.
- Remove the plastic wrap and slide a plastic knife under the glue.
- If it doesn't come away, replace the plastic wrap and leave for another 20 minutes before trying again.

HIGHCHAIRS

To clean

- Wipe with a cake of bathroom soap and cold water on a damp cloth or pantyhose.
- For hardened food, place a damp cloth over the area and leave for 10 minutes. The food will come away when you wipe it down.
- To prevent mould, wipe with a cloth sprayed with ¼ teaspoon of oil of cloves in a 1 litre spray pack of water. Repeat once a month.

ICE BLOCK (FLAVOURED)

On carpet/upholstery

- Remove excess by blotting with paper towel.
- Tightly wring a cloth in white vinegar so it's damp but not wet. Blot over the mark.
- Absorb moisture by covering the area with paper towel. Place a book on top of the paper towel to assist with absorption.
- For a coloured stain, expose to sunlight or UV light. (If using UV light, protect areas around the stain with cardboard.) Check every 2 hours.

On cotton/fabric (not wool)

- Remove excess under the tap using cold water.
- Blot with or soak in white vinegar until the stain is removed.
- Wash according to the fabric. Dry in sunshine.

On wool

- Massage with a small amount of cheap shampoo on your fingertips.
- Rinse in blood-heat (body temperature) water.
- Rinse in 1 teaspoon of cheap hair conditioner and blood-heat water.
- Gently wring and dry flat on a towel in the shade.

ICE CREAM

This is a protein, fat and sugar stain. Remove proteins first.

On carpet/upholstery

- Remove excess by blotting with paper towel.
- Scribble with a cake of bathroom soap run under cold water.
- Scrub with a toothbrush in all directions – north, south, east and west.
- Massage with a couple of drops of dishwashing liquid on your fingertips until the liquid feels like jelly.
- Wipe with a damp cloth.
- Tightly wring a cloth in white vinegar so it's damp but not wet. Blot over the mark.

- Place the vinegar cloth in one hand and a dry cloth in the other and wipe hand over hand, as though stroking a cat, until the stain is removed.
- Absorb moisture by covering the area with paper towel. Place a book on top of the paper towel to assist with absorption.

On cotton/fabric (not wool)

- Remove excess under the tap using cold water.
- Scribble with a cake of bathroom soap run under cold water.
- Massage with a couple of drops of dishwashing liquid on your fingertips until the liquid feels like jelly.
- Rinse in blood-heat (body temperature) water.
- Blot with or soak in white vinegar until the stain is removed.
- Wash according to the fabric. Dry on the clothesline or clothes airer.

On wool

- Massage with a small amount of cheap shampoo on your fingertips.
- Rinse in blood-heat (body temperature) water.
- Blot with or soak in white vinegar.
- Rinse in 1 teaspoon of cheap hair conditioner and blood-heat water.
- Gently wring and dry flat on a towel in the shade.

JUICE

NOTE: Apple, blackcurrant, orange, pineapple and rosehip juice are treated differently – see the relevant entry.

On carpet/upholstery

- Remove excess by blotting with paper towel.
- Tightly wring a cloth in white vinegar so it's damp but not wet. Blot over the mark.
- Absorb moisture by covering the area with paper towel. Place a book on top of the paper towel to assist with absorption.

On cotton/fabric

- Remove excess under the tap using cold water.
- Blot with or soak in white vinegar. Alternatively, soak with ½ lid of *Vanish NapiSan Oxi Action Sensitive Powder* in a 9 litre bucket of water for 30 minutes. Don't use on wool, silk or leather.
- Wash according to the fabric. Dry on the clothesline or clothes airer.

On stone

- Remove excess by blotting with paper towel.
- Scrub with dishwashing liquid on a toothbrush.
- Wipe with a damp cloth.
- If stubborn, mix plaster of Paris and water to the consistency of peanut butter.

- To each cup of mixture, add 1 teaspoon of dishwashing liquid.
- Spread 5 mm to 1 cm thick over the stain.
- Allow to dry completely. If it feels cold on the back of your hand, it's not dry.
- When dry, brush away

LOLLIES

On carpet/upholstery

- Remove excess by lifting with a plastic comb or by blotting with paper towel.
- Tightly wring a cloth in white vinegar so it's damp but not wet. Blot over the mark. If the stain contains liquorice, leave for 10 minutes.
- To remove colouring, expose to sunlight or UV light. (If using UV light, protect areas around the stain with cardboard.) Check every 2 hours.
- In all cases, absorb moisture by covering the area with paper towel. Place a book on top of the paper towel to assist with absorption.

On cotton/fabric

- Remove excess under the tap using cold water.
- Blot with or soak in white vinegar. If the stain contains liquorice, leave for 10 minutes.Hang in sunshine until the stain fades before washing.
- Wash according to the fabric. Dry on the clothesline or clothes airer.

LOTION

(see OINTMENT)

MEDICINES

Children's medicines often contain colourants. Red pigments from cherries can be difficult to remove.

On carpet/upholstery

- Remove excess by blotting with paper towel.
- Scribble with a cake of bathroom soap run under cold water.
- Massage with a couple of drops of dishwashing liquid on your fingertips until the liquid feels like jelly.
- Wipe with a damp cloth until the dishwashing liquid is removed.
- If there's residue, scrub with 2 drops of glycerine on a toothbrush. Leave for 90 minutes. Tightly wring a cloth in white vinegar, fold the cloth flat and polish out the glycerine without pushing it into the back of the carpet or upholstery.
- To remove colouring, follow instructions above then expose to sunlight or UV light. (If using UV light, protect areas around the stain with cardboard.) Check every 2 hours.
- In all cases, absorb moisture by covering the area with paper towel. Place a book on top of the paper towel to assist with absorption.

On cotton/fabric

- Remove excess under the tap using cold water.
- Scribble with a cake of bathroom soap run under cold water.
- Massage with a couple of drops of dishwashing liquid on your fingertips until the liquid feels like jelly.
- If there's residue, scrub with 2 drops of glycerine on a toothbrush. Leave for 90 minutes. Blot with white vinegar and hang in sunshine until the stain fades before washing.
- Wash according to the fabric. Dry on the clothesline or clothes airer.

MILK

(see BREAST MILK. Although their contents are slightly different, the technique to remove milk and breast milk is the same.)

MOULD

On carpet/upholstery (not leather/suede)

- Remove excess by vacuuming.
- Mix ¼ teaspoon of oil of cloves in 1 litre of water in a spray pack. Lightly spray over the area.
- Sprinkle with uniodised salt.
- Scrub with a clean broom.
- Vacuum.

On cotton/fabric

- Remove excess under the tap using cold water.
- Soak in ½ lid of *Vanish NapiSan Oxi Action Sensitive Powder* and 9 litres of blood-heat (body temperature) water for 20 minutes. Don't use on wool, silk or leather.
- If mould remains, add 1 kg of uniodised salt to a 9 litre bucket of water. Soak fabric overnight.
- Remove, gently wring but don't rinse, and hang in the shade to dry. A salt crust will form.
- Brush the salt off and the mould will come off with it.
- Wash according to the fabric. Dry on the clothesline or clothes airer.

On delicates

- Wipe with methylated spirits on a cloth.
- Add 1 cup of uniodised salt to a 9 litre bucket of blood-heat (body temperature) water.
- Immerse the garments and soak overnight (salt water won't damage delicates).
- Gently wring but don't rinse the items and hang them up to dry (in the shade is best). A salty crust will form.
- When dry, brush the crust off with a soft brush and the mould will come away with it.
- Rinse in 1 teaspoon of cheap shampoo and blood-heat water.
- Gently wring and dry flat on a towel in the shade.

On leather

- Mix ¼ teaspoon of oil of cloves in a 250 ml bottle of baby oil. Shake the bottle and re-label it.
- Wipe the mixture with a cloth in even, parallel strokes across the entire panel of leather.

On polyester satin

- Aim a hair dryer over the mould until it warms.
- Rub a clothes brush in the direction of the watery-looking part of the fabric.
- If any mould remains, cover with uniodised salt and brush backwards and forwards with a clothes brush. The salt does the cleaning.

On silicone

- If mould is on the surface of the silicone, sprinkle with bicarb, spray with white vinegar and scrub with a toothbrush.
- If mould has penetrated the silicone, you may have to replace it. Test first by spraying with ¼ teaspoon of oil of cloves in 1 litre of water in a spray pack. Spray over the area and leave for 24 hours.
- To replace silicone, remove the old silicone with a special silicone remover or a very sharp knife. Then replace with new silicone or candle wax.

MYSTERY STAINS

If you don't know what the stain is, use this guide.

Proteins

- These have a dark ring around the edge and include blood, seeds, nuts, meat, cheese, milk, other dairy and fish.
- To remove, use cold water and scribble with a cake of bathroom soap. On fabrics, rub the fabric against itself to loosen the stain. Don't use blood-heat (body temperature) or hot water, or you'll set the stain.

Carbohydrates

- Stains are darker in the centre, lighter around the edge and feel stiff. The causes include sugar, fruit, fruit juice, cakes, biscuits, lollies, soft drink, alcohol, honey, many plants, starches (such as potato, rice, corn, ground corn), wheat-based products (pasta, couscous, etc.), floury grain foods and wallpaper paste.
- To remove sugar stains, use blood-heat (body temperature) water and scribble with a cake of bathroom soap. Rub the fabric against itself to loosen the stain.
- To remove starchy stains, use cold water and scribble with a cake of bathroom soap. Rub the fabric against itself to loosen the stain. If in doubt, use cold water first.

Fats/oils

▓ Stains spread evenly across a surface, feel greasy between your fingers and, if you wash the stained garment, continue to spread. This is why a greasy chip mark on your T-shirt gets bigger every time you wash it. Stains include cooking oils (lighter in colour) and mechanical oils (darker in colour and more viscous).

▓ To remove lighter oils, massage with dishwashing liquid on your fingertips until the liquid feels like jelly. This means the oil has been emulsified and is water soluble. Wipe with a damp cloth or rinse under blood-heat water.

▓ For darker or thicker oils, such as engine grease, use baby oil to dilute the stain before emulsifying with dishwashing liquid.

Pigments

▓ These include ink, paint, dye, rust and oxide; each requires a different solution.

▓ For ink stains, place rotten milk solids over the stain (leave full cream milk in the sun to rot). The ink will be absorbed into the solids. Alternatively, rub with white spirits on a cotton bud.

▓ Permanent pen markers contain their own solvent, so write over the mark with the same pen and, while it's wet, wipe with white spirits on a cotton bud.

▓ For children's or artists' watercolour paint, blot with water on a cloth until removed.

- For water-based paint, use methylated spirits on a cotton bud or cotton ball.
- For oil-based paint, use white spirits or turpentine on a cotton bud or cotton ball.
- For fresh vinyl-based or acrylic paint, blot with a couple of drops of dishwashing liquid on a damp, cold cloth.
- For old vinyl-based or acrylic paint, blot with methylated spirits on a cloth.
- To remove rust from hard surfaces, use proprietary products *CLR* or *Ranex* and always wear rubber gloves when using. Don't get *CLR* or *Ranex* on your skin because they can cause irritation. To remove rust from absorbent surfaces, use lemon juice and salt.
- For a vegetable-based stain, wipe with white vinegar on a cloth.
- For an oxide stain, wipe with 2 drops of glycerine on a cloth and remove any remaining colour by exposing the stain to UV light. Protect the area around the UV light with cardboard.

Resins

- These include sap, chewing gum, shellac, silicone, wax and glue; they feel sticky to touch.
- For plant-based resins, such as tree sap, wipe with glycerine or tea tree oil.
- The solvent for shellac is methylated spirits applied with a cloth.
- For super glue, remove with super glue remover or acetone.

- For craft and PVA glues (which go on white and dry clear), use steam.
- For two-part epoxy glues (e.g. *Araldite*), remove with acetone.
- For gums and paper glues, wipe with a damp cloth.
- For contact adhesives, remove with tea tree oil.
- Glues used in children's crafts are made with carbohydrates, so use blood-heat (body temperature) water and a cake of bathroom soap and scribble over the stain.
- To remove silicone, carefully cut it off with a utility knife. Remove residue by wiping with pantyhose dipped in kerosene.

NAIL POLISH

Nail polish is like a magnet for little ones. It's best to store it away from young hands but if you do spill it, this is how to remove it.

On carpet/upholstery

- Wrap a fine-toothed metal comb in a tissue so the teeth come through the tissue. Don't use a plastic comb because acetone, the solvent, will melt it.
- Wedge the comb underneath the stain and rub the stain with acetone on a cotton ball. Acetone can affect carpet so make sure it doesn't penetrate the base.
- Replace the tissue when wet.
- It's a slow process and may need to be repeated a few times.

- To remove the smell of acetone, wipe with equal parts methylated spirits or white vinegar and water on a tightly wrung cloth.
- Absorb moisture by covering the area with paper towel. Place a book on top of the paper towel to assist with absorption.

On cotton/fabric

- Hold a clean cotton ball behind the stain. Wipe with acetone on a cotton ball.
- Rub in a circular motion from the outside to the inside of the stain.
- Repeat until the nail polish colour is removed, replacing the cotton balls as you go.
- Wash according to the fabric. Dry on the clothesline or clothes airer.

On timber

- For a polyurethane finish, wipe over only the nail polish with acetone on a cotton bud. Work quickly, using as little pressure and acetone as possible.
- When the colour is removed, wipe with white vinegar on a cloth.
- If the surface is dulled, polish with a little Brasso on a cloth.
- For oil-based varnish, shellac or wax-based surfaces, use the same technique but polish with a little beeswax rather than Brasso.
- Acetone can affect acrylic surfaces so you may need to reapply the acrylic.

On upholstery (not leather)

- Blot with acetone on a cotton bud.
- When removed, wipe with a little methylated spirits or white vinegar on a cotton bud. Do this quickly because acetone can damage the upholstery.

NAPPY (CLOTH)

Nappy buckets should have a tightly fitting lid and be changed regularly. To deter mould, wipe over the edge with ¼ teaspoon of oil of cloves in 1 litre spray pack of water.

To clean

- Fill one bucket ¾ full of water and add Shannon's nappy soaker. Make this by mixing 1 teaspoon of 3 per cent hydrogen peroxide and 1 teaspoon of homemade laundry detergent (1 tablespoon of pure soap flakes, juice of 1 lemon and 2 tablespoons of bicarb in a large jar. Add 2 cups of warm water and mix well.)
- Fill a second bucket with hot water and add 1 teaspoon of tea tree oil.
- Shake the solids from the nappy into the toilet.
- Rinse the nappy under water.
- Place nappies in the first bucket and leave for 12 hours.
- Place nappies in the second bucket and leave for 20 minutes.
- Wash in the washing machine with hot water and 1 teaspoon of *Vanish NapiSan Oxi Action Sensitive Powder* or ¼ cup bicarb.

- Add ½ cup of white vinegar to the fabric conditioner slot.
- Dry in the sun.

For wool nappies

- Clean with 1 teaspoon of cheap shampoo in a 9 litre bucket of water.
- Rinse in water and dry in sunshine.
- To replace lanolin, place 1 teaspoon of lanolin in a microwave-safe dish (glass or ceramic, not plastic) with 1 cup of hot water and heat until the lanolin melts. Wring the wool nappies in the solution and dry in sunshine.

NAPPY RASH CREAM

On carpet/upholstery

- Remove excess by lifting with a plastic comb or by blotting with paper towel.
- For lanolin-based cream, massage with a couple of drops of dishwashing liquid on your fingertips until the liquid feels like jelly.
- Mix 1 teaspoon of tea tree oil with 1 cup of cold water and wipe on with a cloth.
- For zinc-based cream, sprinkle with talcum powder and scrub with pantyhose first.
- Mix 1 teaspoon of tea tree oil with 1 cup of cold water and wipe on with a cloth.
- Absorb moisture by covering the area with paper towel. Place a book on top of the paper towel to assist with absorption.

NUTELLA

The stain is from protein, fat and sugar.

On carpet/upholstery

- Remove excess by lifting with a plastic comb or by blotting with paper towel.
- Scribble with a cake of bathroom soap run under cold water.
- Massage with a couple of drops of dishwashing liquid on your fingertips until the liquid feels like jelly.
- Wipe with a damp cloth until the dishwashing liquid is removed.
- Tightly wring a cloth in white vinegar so it's damp but not wet. Blot over the mark.
- Absorb moisture by covering the area with paper towel. Place a book on top of the paper towel to assist with absorption.

On cotton/fabric

- Remove excess under the tap using cold water.
- Scribble with a cake of bathroom soap run under cold water.
- Massage with a couple of drops of dishwashing liquid on your fingertips until the liquid feels like jelly.
- Blot with or soak in white vinegar.
- Wash according to the fabric. Dry on the clothesline or clothes airer.

OINTMENT

On carpet/upholstery

- Remove excess by lifting with a plastic comb or by blotting with paper towel.
- For water-based ointments, scribble with a cake of bathroom soap run under blood-heat (body temperature) water. Massage with your fingertips until the stain is loosened. Wipe with a damp cloth. Repeat, if needed.
- For grey staining, massage with a couple of drops of dishwashing liquid on your fingertips until the liquid feels like jelly. Wipe with a damp cloth until the dishwashing liquid is removed.
- For antibacterial ointments, combine 1 teaspoon of grated bathroom soap, 1 teaspoon of dishwashing liquid and 1 tablespoon of boiling water and mix until the soap dissolves. Massage 2 drops of the solution into the stain using your fingertips until the solution feels like jelly. Wipe with a cold, damp cloth followed by a dry cloth hand over hand, as though stroking a cat.
- For wax-based ointments, mix 2 drops of tea tree oil and 2 drops of dishwashing liquid and massage with your fingertips until the liquid feels like jelly. Wipe with a cold, damp cloth. Repeat, if needed.
- For liniment (alcohol-based), wring a cloth in white vinegar, place over the stain and stand or sit on it for 5 seconds. Remove.

■ In all cases, absorb moisture by covering the area with paper towel. Place a book on top of the paper towel to assist with absorption.

On cotton/fabric (not wool)

■ Remove excess under the tap using blood-heat (body temperature) water.

■ For water-based ointments, scribble with a cake of bathroom soap. Massage with your fingertips until the stain is loosened.

■ For grey staining, massage with a couple of drops of dishwashing liquid on your fingertips until the liquid feels like jelly.

■ For antibacterial ointments, combine 1 teaspoon of grated bathroom soap, 1 teaspoon of dishwashing liquid and 1 tablespoon of boiling water. Allow the mixture to dissolve. Massage 2 drops of the solution into the stain with your fingertips until the solution feels like jelly.

■ For wax-based ointments, mix 2 drops of tea tree oil with 2 drops of dishwashing liquid and massage with your fingertips until the liquid feels like jelly.

■ For liniment (alcohol-based), blot with or soak in white vinegar.

■ In all cases, wash according to the fabric. Dry on the clothesline or clothes airer.

ORANGE JUICE

On carpet/upholstery

- For a fresh stain, remove excess by blotting with paper towel. Tightly wring a cloth in white vinegar and blot over the mark.
- For an old stain, brush the surface with 2 drops of glycerine on a toothbrush. Tightly wring a cloth in white vinegar, fold the cloth flat and polish out the glycerine without pushing it into the back of the carpet or upholstery.
- To remove dye, expose to sunlight or UV light. (If using UV light, protect areas around the stain with cardboard.) Check every 2 hours.
- In all cases, absorb moisture by covering the area with paper towel. Place a book on top of the paper towel to assist with absorption.

On cotton/fabric (not wool)

- Remove excess under the tap using cold water.
- Blot with or soak in white vinegar until the stain is removed. Alternatively, soak in ½ lid of *Vanish NapiSan Oxi Action Sensitive Powder* and 9 litres of water for 20 minutes. Don't use on wool, silk or leather.
- Wash according to the fabric. Dry on the clothesline or clothes airer in sunshine.

On wool

- Blot with or soak in white vinegar on a cloth.
- Massage with a little cheap shampoo on your fingertips.

- Rinse in blood-heat (body temperature) water.
- Rinse in 1 teaspoon of cheap hair conditioner and blood-heat water.
- Gently wring and dry flat on a towel in the shade. If there's an orange residue, dry in sunshine.

PAINT

On carpet/upholstery

- Remove excess by lifting with a plastic comb or by blotting with paper towel. Try not to spread it.
- For children's and artists' water colour paint, blot with water on a cloth until removed.
- For fresh vinyl-based or acrylic paint, blot with a couple of drops of dishwashing liquid on a damp, cold cloth.
- For old vinyl-based or acrylic paint, soak a cloth with methylated spirits and place it over the stain. Cover in plastic wrap. Leave for 1 hour.
- For water-based paint, use methylated spirits on a cotton bud or cotton ball.
- For oil-based paint, use white spirits or turpentine on a cotton bud or cotton ball.
- In all cases, absorb moisture by covering the area with paper towel. Place a book on top of the paper towel to assist with absorption.

On cotton/fabric

- For children's and artists' water colour paint, rinse off using cold water. If stubborn, rub the fabric with 2 drops of dishwashing liquid until removed.
- For vinyl-based or acrylic paint, place a clean cotton ball behind the stain, then wipe with methylated spirits on a cotton ball.
- For water-based paint, use methylated spirits on a cotton bud or cotton ball.
- For oil-based paint, place a clean cotton ball behind the stain, then wipe with white spirits or turpentine on a cotton ball.
- In all cases, wipe in a circular motion from the outside to the inside of the stain.
- If stubborn, soak in the appropriate solvent.
- In all cases, wash according to the fabric. Dry on the clothesline or clothes airer.

PEANUT BUTTER

On carpet/upholstery

- Remove excess by lifting with a plastic comb or by blotting with paper towel.
- Massage with a couple of drops of dishwashing liquid on your fingertips until the liquid feels like jelly.
- Wipe with a damp cloth until dishwashing liquid is removed.
- Absorb moisture by covering the area with paper towel. Place a book on top of the paper towel to assist with absorption.

On cotton/fabric

- Remove excess by lifting with a plastic comb.
- Massage with a couple of drops of dishwashing liquid on your fingertips until the liquid feels like jelly.
- Rinse with blood-heat (body temperature) water.
- Wash according to the fabric. Dry on the clothesline or clothes airer.

On granite/marble/timber

- Mix plaster of Paris and water to the consistency of peanut butter.
- To each cup of mixture, add 1 teaspoon of dishwashing liquid.
- Spread 5 mm to 1 cm thick over the stain.
- Allow to dry completely. If it feels cold on the back of your hand, it's not dry.
- When dry, brush off with a broom or brush.

PEAS

On carpet/upholstery

- Remove excess by lifting with a plastic comb or by blotting with paper towel.
- Brush with 2 drops of glycerine on a toothbrush (don't push it into the backing). Leave for 90 minutes.
- For a green stain, expose to sunlight or UV light. (If using UV light, protect areas around the stain with cardboard.) Check every 2 hours.

- Wipe with a damp cloth.
- Absorb moisture by covering the area with paper towel. Place a book on top of the paper towel to assist with absorption.

On cotton/fabric

- Remove excess under the tap using cold water.
- Wipe with 2 drops of glycerine on a cloth. Leave for 90 minutes.
- Blot with or soak in white vinegar until the stain is removed.
- Wash according to the fabric. Dry on the clothesline or clothes airer.

On timber

- For a polyurethane finish, polish with equal parts glycerine and talcum powder on a cloth.
- For a shellac finish, wipe with beeswax on a cloth.
- To remove a green stain, expose to sunlight or UV light. (If using UV light, protect areas around the stain with cardboard.) Check every 2 hours.

PEN MARKS

There are several types of ink used in pens. Test the solvent using a cotton bud.

Ballpoint pen/bottled ink (non-gel)

On carpet/upholstery (not leather)

- Rot some full cream milk in the sun.
- Place the rotten milk solids on the stain and rub in circles with your hands.
- When the ink is absorbed, wipe away the milk solids with a damp cloth.
- Scribble the stain with a cake of bathroom soap run under blood-heat (body temperature) water.
- Wipe with a damp cloth.
- Absorb moisture by covering the area with paper towel. Place a book on top of the paper towel to assist with absorption.
- Alternatively, wipe with white spirits on a cloth or cotton bud.
- Sprinkle with talcum powder.
- When dry, vacuum.

On cotton/fabric

- Rot some full cream milk in the sun. Place the rotten milk solids over the stain. For red ink, wipe with white spirits on a cotton ball first.
- Leave until the ink is absorbed into the solids.
- Remove the solids under cold water.
- Scribble with a cake of bathroom soap run under blood-heat (body temperature) water. Rub the fabric against itself using your hands.

- Wash according to the fabric. Dry on the clothesline or clothes airer.

On leather

- Wipe over the mark with white spirits on a cotton bud. If there's a watermark, wipe with white spirits in even, parallel strokes over the entire panel of leather.
- Sprinkle evenly with talcum powder.
- When dry, brush with a soft brush.
- Wipe with leather conditioner. Make your own by placing 1 teaspoon of beeswax, 1 teaspoon of lavender oil and 1 teaspoon of lemon oil on a soft cotton cloth, such as an old T-shirt. Place in the microwave in a microwave-safe dish. Microwave on high in 10-second bursts until the beeswax melts. After using it, place the cloth in a zip-lock bag and store in the freezer ready to use again.

On stone

- Rot some full cream milk in the sun.
- Place the milk solids over the stain.
- Leave until the ink bleeds into the solids.
- Remove with a damp cloth.

On timber

- Wipe with white spirits on a cotton bud.
- Alternatively, rot some full cream milk in the sun. Place the solids over the stain until the ink is absorbed.
- In both cases, wipe with a damp cloth.

Felt pen

- For children's felt pen, wipe with methylated spirits on a cotton bud or cotton ball.
- For adults' felt pen, wipe with white spirits on a cotton bud or cotton ball. Work from the outside to the inside of the stain.

Gel pen

- A gel pen has a ball of clear liquid at the end of the gel in the plastic tube.
- Wipe with methylated spirits on a cotton bud.

Liquid marker

On carpet/upholstery

- The solvent is either methylated spirits or white spirits.
- Test by wiping with both solvents separately on a cotton bud. If marker colour comes away, that's the solvent.
- Wipe the solvent in circles on a cotton ball until removed. You may need to use several cotton balls.
- Sprinkle with talcum powder.
- When dry, vacuum.

On cotton/fabric

- The solvent is either methylated spirits or white spirits.
- Test by wiping with both solvents separately on a cotton bud. If marker colour comes away, that's the solvent.

- Blot with or soak in the solvent.
- Wash according to the fabric. Dry on the clothesline or clothes airer.

On timber

- Write over the mark using the same pen.
- Wipe with white spirits on a cotton bud.

Permanent marker

- Permanent marker contains its own solvent, so draw over the mark with the same permanent marker.
- Wipe with white spirits on a cotton bud or cotton ball.
- Sprinkle with talcum powder.

Texta

- Wipe with methylated spirits on a cotton bud or cotton ball.

Whiteboard marker

- Wipe with methylated spirits on a cotton bud or cotton ball.

PINEAPPLE/PINEAPPLE JUICE

On carpet/upholstery

- Remove excess by blotting with paper towel.
- Tightly wring a cloth in white vinegar so it's damp but not wet. Blot over the mark.
- If staining remains, spray with *Vanish Preen Oxi Action Carpet Stain Remover.*

- Leave for 30 minutes.
- When dry, vacuum.

On cotton/fabric

- Remove excess under the tap using cold water.
- Blot with or soak in white vinegar.
- For brown marks, wipe with 2 drops of glycerine on a cloth. Leave for 90 minutes.
- Wash according to the fabric. Dry on the clothesline or clothes airer.

PLASTICINE

On carpet/upholstery

- Remove excess by lifting with a plastic comb.
- Massage with 2 drops of dishwashing liquid and 2 drops of lavender oil on your fingertips until the mixture feels like jelly.
- Wipe with a damp cloth until dishwashing liquid is removed.
- Absorb moisture by covering the area with paper towel. Place a book on top of the paper towel to assist with absorption.

On cotton/fabric

- Remove excess under the tap using blood-heat (body temperature) water.
- Massage with 2 drops of dishwashing liquid and 2 drops of lavender oil on your fingertips until the mixture feels like jelly.

- Wash according to the fabric. Dry on the clothesline or clothes airer.

PLAY DOUGH

On carpet/upholstery

- Allow to dry. Scrub with a stiff brush and vacuum as you scrub.
- Scrub with a little uniodised salt on pantyhose or a toothbrush.
- For large areas, sprinkle with unprocessed wheat bran and scrub.
- To remove colour, wipe with white vinegar on a cloth and expose to sunlight or UV light. (If using UV light, protect areas around the stain with cardboard.) Check every 2 hours.
- Vacuum thoroughly.
- Repeat until removed.

On cotton/fabric

- Allow to dry.
- Scrub with a little uniodised salt on pantyhose or a toothbrush.
- To remove colour, blot with or soak in white vinegar. Hang in sunshine until the stain fades before washing.
- Wash according to the fabric. Dry on the clothesline or clothes airer.

POO

It depends what your baby or toddler is eating. A baby's digestion doesn't easily break down colourants. The first time they eat beetroot or strawberries creates a big surprise in the nappy. After washing, hang clothes or nappies in sunshine to fade stains.

On carpet/upholstery

- Remove excess by lifting with a plastic comb or by blotting with paper towel.
- If there are colourants, wipe across the surface with 2 drops of glycerine on a toothbrush (don't push into the backing). Leave for 90 minutes.
- Scribble with a cake of bathroom soap run under cold water.
- Wipe with a damp cloth.
- Massage with a couple of drops of dishwashing liquid on your fingertips until the liquid feels like jelly.
- Wipe with a damp cloth until the dishwashing liquid is removed.
- Absorb moisture by covering the area with paper towel. Place a book on top of the paper towel to assist with absorption.

On cotton/fabric

- Remove excess under the tap using cold water.
- If there are colourants, wipe with 2 drops of glycerine and leave for 90 minutes.

- Scribble with a cake of bathroom soap run under cold water.
- Massage with a couple of drops of dishwashing liquid on your fingertips until the liquid feels like jelly.
- Rinse using cold water.
- Alternatively, soak overnight in a bucket of cold water and ¼ cup of bicarb.
- In both cases, wash according to the fabric. Dry in sunshine to fade remaining stains.

PRAM

To clean plastic

- Mix 1 teaspoon of dishwashing liquid with 1 litre of water in a spray pack.
- Spray the mixture over the pram and scrub with a brush.
- Rinse with water on a cloth. Dry in sunshine.

To clean canvas

- Mix 1 kg of uniodised salt and ¼ teaspoon of oil of cloves in a 9 litre bucket of water. Allow to dissolve.
- Scrub with the mixture using a nylon brush.
- Leave in the sun until dry, then brush off the salt.

To clean aluminium

- Wipe with a damp tea bag in the toe of pantyhose.

PUMPKIN

On carpet/upholstery

- Remove excess by lifting with a plastic comb or by blotting with paper towel.
- Tightly wring a cloth in white vinegar so it's damp but not wet. Blot over the mark.
- To remove an orange stain, expose to sunlight or UV light. (If using UV light, protect areas around the stain with cardboard.) Check every 2 hours.
- Absorb moisture by covering the area with paper towel. Place a book on top of the paper towel to assist with absorption.

On cotton/fabric (not wool)

- Remove excess under the tap using cold water.
- Blot with or soak in white vinegar until the stain is removed.
- Wash according to the fabric. Dry in sunshine.

On wool

- Place equal parts white vinegar and cold water on a cloth and wring tightly so it's damp but not wet. Blot over the mark.
- If the stain has set, wipe with 2 drops of lavender oil on a cloth. Leave for 20 minutes.
- Wash in 1 teaspoon of cheap shampoo and blood-heat (body temperature) water.
- Rinse in blood-heat water.
- Gently wring and dry flat on a towel in the shade.

ROSEHIP JUICE

This is high in Vitamin C and tannins.

On carpet/upholstery

- Remove excess by blotting with paper towel.
- For an old stain, brush across the surface with 2 drops of glycerine on a toothbrush (don't push into the backing). Leave for 90 minutes. Then follow the instructions below.
- For a fresh stain, sprinkle with bicarb. Leave for 5 minutes, then vacuum.
- Tightly wring a cloth in white vinegar so it's damp but not wet. Blot over the mark.
- Absorb moisture by covering the area with paper towel. Place a book on top of the paper towel to assist with absorption.

On cotton/fabric

- Rinse under the tap using cold water.
- For an old stain, wipe with glycerine and leave for 90 minutes.
- For a fresh stain, blot with or soak in white vinegar.
- In both cases, wash according to the fabric. Dry in sunshine.

SHEEPSKIN

Skeepskin can be washed in the washing machine as long as the temperature of the wash water and rinse water is the same. Rather than laundry detergent, use cheap shampoo.

To clean

- Mix 1 teaspoon of cheap shampoo in a tub of blood-heat (body temperature) water.
- Immerse the sheepskin.
- Gently massage with your hands as though washing your hair.
- Rinse in blood-heat water.
- To prevent stiffening, dry slowly in the shade. Brush regularly with a hairbrush as it's drying.

SNOT

Baby snot on clothes can be difficult to remove.

On cotton/fabric

- Rinse under blood-heat (body temperature) water.
- Scribble with a cake of bathroom soap and blood-heat water.
- Rub the fabric against itself.
- Wash according to the fabric. Dry on the clotheslines or clothes airer.

SOFT DRINK

On carpet/upholstery

- Remove excess by blotting with paper towel.
- Mix equal parts white vinegar and blood-heat (body temperature) water.

- Scrub the mixture with a toothbrush or pantyhose in all directions – north, south, east and west.
- Absorb moisture by covering the area with paper towel. Place a book on top of the paper towel to assist with absorption.
- If there's colour, wipe with white vinegar and expose to sunlight or UV light. (If using UV light, protect areas around the stain with cardboard.) Check every 2 hours.
- If a shadow returns in a couple of weeks, repeat.

On cotton/fabric
- Remove excess under the tap using cold water.
- Blot with or soak in white vinegar and hang in sunshine before washing.
- Wash according to the fabric. Dry in sunshine.

SPAGHETTI SAUCE

(see TOMATO SAUCE)

SPIT-UP MILK

It's common for babies to spit-up partially digested milk, particularly if they have reflux. This spit-up milk contains gastric juices including hydrochloric acid.

On cotton/fabric
- Rinse under cold water.

- Scribble with a cake of bathroom soap and cold water. Formula is more difficult to remove, so scrub over the soap with a stiff brush.
- Wash according to the fabric. Dry in sunshine.

 TIP To protect clothing, wear a rubber-backed towel or cloth over your shoulder to catch the spit-up.

STICKERS

On walls/hard surfaces

- Mix 2 drops of dishwashing liquid in 1 litre of hot water in a spray pack.
- Spray over the sticker and cover with cling wrap. Leave for 1 hour.
- Remove cling wrap and the sticker should come off.
- Alternatively, wring a cloth in white vinegar and place over the area. Leave for 30 minutes.
- Remove and wipe stain with tea tree oil on a cotton ball.
- If stubborn, wipe with eucalyptus oil on paper towel.

SUNSCREEN

On carpet/upholstery

- Remove excess by blotting with paper towel.
- Massage with a couple of drops of dishwashing liquid on your fingertips until the liquid feels like jelly.

- Wipe with a damp cloth until the dishwashing liquid is removed.
- Wipe with 2 drops of glycerine on a toothbrush. Leave for 90 minutes.
- Tightly wring a cloth in white vinegar, fold the cloth flat and polish out the glycerine without pushing it into the back of the carpet or upholstery.
- Absorb moisture by covering the area with paper towel. Place a book on top of the paper towel to assist with absorption.

On cotton/fabric

- Remove excess under the tap using cold water.
- Massage with a couple of drops of dishwashing liquid on your fingertips until the liquid feels like jelly.
- Wipe with 2 drops of glycerine on a toothbrush. Leave for 90 minutes.
- Blot with or soak in white vinegar.
- Wash according to the fabric. Dry on the clothesline or clothes airer.

On plastic in car interior

- Wipe with equal parts glycerine and dishwashing liquid on a cloth.
- Remove with a warm, damp cloth.

SWEET POTATO

On carpet/upholstery

- For cooked sweet potato, remove excess by lifting with a plastic comb. For raw sweet potato, wipe with equal parts glycerine and white vinegar on a cloth first.
- Scribble with a cake of bathroom soap run under cold water.
- Wipe with a damp cloth.
- Absorb moisture by covering the area with paper towel. Place a book on top of the paper towel to assist with absorption.

On cotton/fabric

- For cooked sweet potato, remove excess under the tap using cold water. For raw sweet potato, wipe with equal parts glycerine and white vinegar on a cloth first.
- Scribble with a cake of bathroom soap. Rub the fabric against itself using your hands.
- Wash according to the fabric. Dry on the clothesline or clothes airer.

TOMATO SAUCE

On carpet/upholstery

- Remove excess by lifting with a plastic comb or by blotting with paper towel.
- Tightly wring a cloth in white vinegar so it's damp but not wet. Blot over the mark.

- Absorb moisture by covering the area with paper towel. Place a book on top of the paper towel to assist with absorption.
- For a red stain, expose to sunlight or UV light. (If using UV light, protect areas around the stain with cardboard.) Check every 2 hours.

On cotton/fabric

- Remove excess under the tap using cold water.
- Blot with or soak in white vinegar. For a red stain, hang in sunshine with the stained side facing out before washing. The sun will fade the stain.
- Wash according to the fabric. Dry in sunshine.

On plastic

- Mix 2 drops of glycerine and talcum powder until it forms a paste.
- Wipe on the mixture with a cloth.
- Alternatively, rub uniodised salt and lemon juice into the plastic and leave in sunshine.

TOOTHPASTE

Remove as soon as possible because it can bleach surfaces.

On carpet/upholstery

- Remove excess by lifting with a plastic comb or by blotting with paper towel.

- Tightly wring a cloth in white vinegar so it's damp but not wet. Blot over the mark.
- Absorb moisture by covering the area with paper towel. Place a book on top of the paper towel to assist with absorption.

On timber

- Wipe with water on rolled up pantyhose.
- If the toothpaste has bleached the timber, wipe with a damp tea bag. The tannins in tea draw out the tannins in the timber and replace the colour.

On wool

- Remove excess under the tap using blood-heat (body temperature) water.
- Blot with equal parts white vinegar and water on a cloth.
- Soak in 1 teaspoon of cheap shampoo and blood-heat water for 30 minutes.
- Rinse in blood-heat water.
- Gently wring and dry flat on a towel in the shade.

TOYS

To clean a hard toy

- Mix ¼ teaspoon of tea tree oil and 1 litre of water in a spray pack. Tea tree oil is a great disinfectant and is non-toxic.
- Spray over the toy and wipe with a cloth.

To clean a mouldy rubber toy

- Add ¼ teaspoon of oil of cloves to 4 litres of blood-heat (body temperature) water in a bucket.
- Place the toy in the bucket, squeeze so water gets inside and leave for 2 hours.
- Remove, squeeze out the water and set aside to dry.

To clean a soft toy

- Place inside a plastic bag and put it into the freezer to kill microscopic bugs and dust mites (not the allergen).
- Check the label. Most soft toys can be washed in the washing machine on a gentle cycle. Instead of laundry detergent, use 1 tablespoon of cheap shampoo and 2 drops of tea tree oil to kill dust mites. Place in a delicates bag or pillowcase.
- Don't use the dryer but hang the toys to dry in sunshine.
- Alternatively, after removing from the freezer, mix 1 kg of unprocessed wheat bran and a few drops of white vinegar until the mixture resembles breadcrumbs. Place inside a pillowcase and add the soft toy. Tie off and shake well.
- Remove the toy from the pillowcase and brush with a scrubbing brush.

URINE

On carpet/upholstery

- For fresh stains, remove excess by blotting with paper towel.
- Tightly wring a cloth in white vinegar so it's damp but not wet. Blot over the mark.

- For old stains, turn on a UV light in a darkened room and the urine stains will show up yellow.
- Mark around the stains with a piece of white chalk.
- Blot inside the chalk marks with white vinegar on a cloth.
- Alternatively, for fresh and old stains, fill a bucket with cold water and enough dishwashing liquid to generate a sudsy mix.
- Scrub with only the suds on a toothbrush using as little water as possible.
- Wipe with a damp cloth.
- In all cases, absorb moisture by covering the area with paper towel. Place a book on top of the paper towel to assist with absorption.
- Never soak urine stains because soaking pushes the stain further into the fibres.

On cotton/fabric

- Remove excess under the tap using cold water.
- Blot with or soak in white vinegar.
- Wash according to the fabric. Dry on the clothesline or clothes airer.

On mattress

- Tightly wring a cloth in white vinegar so it's damp but not wet. Blot over the mark.
- Alternatively, add a little dishwashing liquid to water to generate a sudsy mix. Scrub only the suds into the stain with a cloth.

- In both cases, put the mattress in the sun if possible. If not, use paper towel with a book on top to absorb moisture and dry with a hair dryer.
- Neutralise the smell by wiping with lemon juice on a cloth.

On shoes

- Dab the stain with white spirits on a cotton ball.
- Sprinkle with talcum powder inside and outside the shoe.
- Allow to dry and brush out.
- To neutralise the smell, wipe with lemon juice on a cloth.
- Cloth and vinyl shoes can be washed in the washing machine or hand washed and dried in sunshine.

On stone/timber

- If the urine has penetrated, mix plaster of Paris and water to the consistency of peanut butter.
- To each cup of mixture, add 2 teaspoons of white vinegar.
- Spread 5 mm to 1 cm thick over the stain.
- Allow to dry completely. If it feels cold on the back of your hand, it's not dry.
- When dry, brush off with a broom.

VEGEMITE

On carpet/upholstery

- Remove excess by lifting with a plastic comb or by blotting with paper towel.

- Massage with a couple of drops of dishwashing liquid on your fingertips until the liquid feels like jelly.
- Wipe with a damp cloth until the dishwashing liquid is removed.
- Absorb moisture by covering the area with paper towel. Place a book on top of the paper towel to assist with absorption.

On cotton/fabric

- Remove excess under the tap using blood-heat (body temperature) water.
- Massage with a couple of drops of dishwashing liquid on your fingertips until the liquid feels like jelly.
- Wash according to the fabric. Dry on the clothesline or clothes airer.

VOMIT

How to remove vomit stains depends what your baby or toddler was eating.

On carpet/upholstery

- Remove excess by lifting with a plastic comb or by blotting with paper towel.
- Scribble with a cake of bathroom soap run under cold water.
- Massage with a couple of drops of dishwashing liquid on your fingertips until the liquid feels like jelly.
- Wipe with a damp cloth until the dishwashing liquid is removed.

- If the vomit contains bile (pale lime green colour), wipe with equal parts glycerine and dishwashing liquid on a cloth. Wipe with a damp cloth until the dishwashing liquid is removed.
- If there's a watermark, place 1 cup of unprocessed wheat bran in a large bowl. Add drops of white vinegar one at a time, stirring as you go, until the mixture resembles breadcrumbs. It shouldn't be wet. Place the mixture into the toe of pantyhose and tie off tightly. It will be the size of a tennis ball. Rub over the stain until removed.
- To remove the smell, mix 1 tablespoon of lemon juice with 1 litre of water in a spray pack and spray over the area.
- Absorb moisture by covering the area with paper towel. Place a book on top of the paper towel to assist with absorption.

On cotton/fabric

- Remove excess under the tap using cold water.
- For milk vomit, scribble with a cake of bathroom soap as though using a big crayon.
- Massage with a couple of drops of dishwashing liquid on your fingertips until the liquid feels like jelly.
- Blot or soak in white vinegar (to remove hydrochloric acid).
- If there's residue, scrub with 2 drops of glycerine on a toothbrush. Leave for 90 minutes. Blot with white vinegar and hang in sunshine until the stain fades before washing.
- Alternatively, soak in ½ lid of *Vanish NapiSan Oxi Action Sensitive Powder* and 9 litres of hot water for 30 minutes. Don't use on wool or silk. For wool and silk, rinse in 1 teaspoon of cheap shampoo and blood-heat (body temperature) water.

- If it contains bile (pale lime green colour), wipe with equal parts glycerine and dishwashing liquid.
- Wash according to the fabric. Dry on the clothesline or clothes airer.

On mattress

- Remove excess by lifting with a plastic comb or by blotting with paper towel.
- Wipe with a damp cloth.
- To remove the smell, mix 1 tablespoon of lemon juice with 1 litre of water in a spray pack and spray over the mattress.
- If you can, put the mattress in the sun to dry it out and to kill bacteria.
- If you can't get it out into the sunshine, dry with a hair dryer.

VICKS VAPORUB

(See OINTMENT)

WATERMELON

On carpet/upholstery

- Remove excess by lifting with a plastic comb or by blotting with paper towel.
- Tightly wring a cloth in white vinegar so it's damp but not wet. Blot over the mark.
- Sprinkle with a little bicarb. Allow to dry.
- Vacuum.

On cotton/fabric

- Remove excess under the tap using cold water.
- Blot with or soak in white vinegar.
- Wash according to the fabric. Dry in sunshine.

YELLOWING CLOTHES

On cotton/fabric (not antique/silk/wool)

- For synthetic fibres, dip in methylated spirits and wring out tightly.
- For natural fibres, soak overnight in ½ lid of *Vanish NapiSan Oxi Action Sensitive Powder* and 9 litres of blood-heat (body temperature) to hot water. Don't use on wool or silk.
- In both cases, wash according to the fabric. Dry in sunshine.

On wool

- Soak with 1 teaspoon of cheap shampoo and 1 tablespoon of 3 per cent hydrogen peroxide in 9 litres of blood-heat (body temperature) water for 20 minutes. Place a dinner plate on top to keep item immersed.
- Rinse in blood-heat water.
- Gently wring and dry flat on a towel in the shade.

YOGHURT

On carpet/upholstery

- Remove excess by lifting with a plastic comb or by blotting with paper towel.
- Scribble with a cake of bathroom soap run under cold water.
- Wipe with a damp cloth.
- Absorb moisture by covering the area with paper towel. Place a book on top of the paper towel to assist with absorption.

On cotton/fabric

- Remove excess under the tap using cold water.
- Scribble with a cake of bathroom soap run under cold water. Rub the fabric against itself using your hands.
- Wash according to the fabric. Dry on the clothesline or clothes airer.

CHAPTER 9

HOUSEHOLD FORMULAS

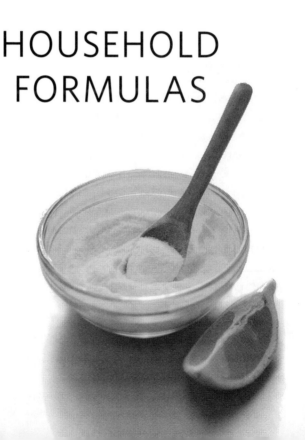

ACID-FREE DRAWER LINERS

- Fill a spray pack with warm water, add 1 tea bag and allow to sit for 3 minutes. Remove the tea bag and add 2 drops of oil of cloves and your favourite perfume or essential oil to the bottle.
- Spray the mixture over acid-free paper (available from newsagencies and removalists).
- Allow the paper to dry, cut to size and place in drawers and cupboards. Replace each year.

BRAN BALL

(can be used on upholstery, fabric, suede)
- Put 1 cup of unprocessed wheat bran in a bowl and add white vinegar, 1 drop at a time, until the mixture resembles breadcrumbs – it should be clumping but not wet.
- Place the mixture into the toe of pantyhose and tie tightly. Rub the pantyhose across the stained surface like an eraser.
- The bran ball can be reused again and again. Store in a zip-lock bag in the freezer. Add drops of white vinegar to re-moisten.

CARPET CLEANER

(for steam cleaning)
- Carpet steam-cleaning machines can be hired at supermarkets. They come with a bottle of cleaning chemicals.

- Use only half the amount the manufacturer suggests and top up with 2 tablespoons of bicarb, 2 tablespoons of white vinegar, 2 tablespoons of methylated spirits, 2 teaspoons of glycerine and 2 teaspoons of eucalyptus oil.
- This solution is also a great multi-purpose spot cleaner. Store in a 1 litre spray pack and use as needed.

COCKROACH DETERRENT

- Mix 1 cup of uniodised salt, 1 teaspoon of lavender oil and 1 litre of water in a spray pack.
- Spray the solution around doors, windows, drains, air vents and other areas where cockroaches lurk. Re-spray when you see cockroaches – more often during summer.

FURNITURE POLISH/LEATHER CONDITIONER

- Place 1 teaspoon of beeswax, 1 teaspoon of lavender oil and 1 teaspoon of lemon oil on a soft cotton cloth, such as an old T-shirt.
- Place in the microwave in a microwave-safe dish. Microwave on high in 10-second bursts until the beeswax melts.
- When it cools, use on leather and timber.
- After use, place the cloth in a zip-lock bag and store in the freezer, ready to use again.

GENERAL CLEANER FOR CARPET

- Mix 2 tablespoons of bicarb, 2 tablespoons of white vinegar, 2 tablespoons of methylated spirits, 2 teaspoons of glycerine, 2 teaspoons of eucalyptus oil, 2 teaspoons of dishwashing liquid and 1 litre of water in a spray pack. Lightly spray over carpet, then wipe with a damp cloth.

GLYCERINE SOLUTION

(to remove tannin stains)
- Mix 2 tablespoons of glycerine with 2 cups of water and place in a 1 litre spray pack.
- Lightly mist over areas. Leave for 90 minutes. Wipe off with a damp cloth.

HARD SURFACE CLEANER

- Combine 1 teaspoon of lavender oil, 1 cup of white vinegar and 1 litre of water in a spray pack. Shake well before use.
- Lightly mist over hard surfaces, then wipe surfaces with a clean cloth.
- Don't use this cleaner on marble because white vinegar is an acid and will eat into marble.

INSECTICIDE SPRAY

- Mix 4 teaspoons of dried mint or 8 teaspoons of freshly chopped mint with 1 litre of boiling water in a spray pack.
- Let it sit for 15 minutes. Spray as needed.

LAUNDRY DETERGENT FOR DELICATES AND SOFT WOOLLENS

- Mix ½ cup of pure soap flakes, ¼ cup of cheap shampoo, 2 teaspoons of bicarb and 2 teaspoons of white vinegar in a clean laundry detergent bottle. Add 2 litres of water, shake, and it's ready to use. Don't forget to re-label the bottle.
- Add fragrance if desired, such as 2 teaspoons of lavender oil, but be careful adding eucalyptus oil because it strips colour and oils from fabric.
- Add ½ teaspoon of tea tree oil to the mixture to make it disinfectant and antiviral.
- For a regular size, lightly soiled load, use 1 tablespoon of this mixture for a top loader and ½ tablespoon for a front loader.

LAUNDRY DETERGENT FOR SENSITIVE SKIN

- Combine 1 tablespoon of pure soap flakes, the juice of 1 lemon and 2 tablespoons of bicarb in a large jar. Add 2 cups of warm water and mix well. Label the jar.
- For a regular size, lightly soiled load, use 1 tablespoon of this mixture for a top loader and ½ tablespoon for a front loader.

 TIP Use white vinegar in the fabric softener slot of the washing machine. It will remove excess soap.

LEMON OIL

▦ Place lemon zest (grate the peel) on plastic wrap and leave on a sunny windowsill. The oil will leach from the peel onto the plastic. Store in a small vial.

MATERNITY CLOTHES

▦ To extend a shirt, cut the side seams and attach a matching fabric tab with a button. Wear a jacket over the top to cover the seams.

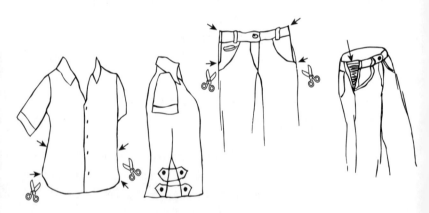

▦ To add elastic to a pair of pants, cut the side seams and insert a V-shaped piece of elastic into each cut. The insert can be removed after pregnancy and you can still wear your favourite jeans.

MOULD REMOVER FOR HARD SURFACES

- Mix ¼ teaspoon of oil of cloves in a 1 litre spray pack of water.
- Spray and leave for 24 hours before respraying. Wipe surfaces with a clean cloth.

NAPPY FOLDING

- Most people fold DBAC, but this makes for too many folds and thick edges against the baby's skin. If you fold ACDB, you are left with more smooth fabric against the baby.

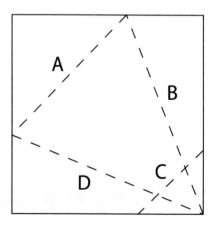

NAPPY SOAKER – SHANNON'S RECIPE

- Fill a bucket ¾ full of water and mix 1 teaspoon of 3 per cent hydrogen peroxide and 1 teaspoon of laundry detergent for sensitive skin (1 tablespoon of pure soap flakes, juice of 1 lemon and 2 tablespoons of bicarb in a large jar. Add 2 cups of warm water and mix well.) Stir through.

PRE-WASH LAUNDRY SPRAY

- Mix 2 tablespoons of methylated spirits, 2 teaspoons of lavender oil, 1 teaspoon of tea tree oil, 2 teaspoons of glycerine, 1 teaspoon of dishwashing liquid and 500 ml of warm water in a spray pack.
- Shake and lightly mist as needed.

SURFACE SPRAY

- Mix 1 teaspoon of lavender oil with 1 litre of water in a spray pack. Use on hard surfaces.

INDEX